Perianesthesia
Patient Care *for*

UNCOMMON DISEASES

Perianesthesia Patient Care *for*

UNCOMMON DISEASES

Joseph Anthony Joyce, CRNA, BS

Staff Certified Registered Nurse Anesthetist
Moses Cone Health System
Wesley Long Community Hospital
Greensboro, North Carolina

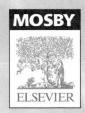

MOSBY

ELSEVIER

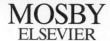

MOSBY
ELSEVIER

11830 Westline Industrial Drive
St. Louis, Missouri 63146

Perianesthesia Patient Care for Uncommon Diseases
ISBN-13: 978-0-323-04568-1

Notice

Knowledge and best practice in this field are constantly changing. As new
research and experience broaden our knowledge, changes in practice, treatment
and drug therapy may become necessary or appropriate. Readers are advised
to check the most current information provided (i) on procedures featured
or (ii) by the manufacturer of each product to be administered, to verify the
recommended dose or formula, the method and duration of administration,
and contraindications. It is the responsibility of the practitioner, relying on
their own experience and knowledge of the patient, to make diagnoses, to
determine dosages and the best treatment for each individual patient, and to
take all appropriate safety precautions. To the fullest extent of the law, neither
the Publisher nor the Author assumes any liability for any injury and/or damage
to persons or property arising out or related to any use of the material contained
in this book.

The Publisher

ISBN-13: 978-0-323-04568-1

Editor: Kristin Geen
Managing Editor: Tamara Myers
Senior Developmental Editor: Laura Selkirk
Developmental Editor: Tina Kaemmerer
Publishing Services Manager: Jeffrey Patterson
Project Manager: Mary G. Stueck
Designer: Andrea Lutes

Printed in the United States of America

Last digit is the print number: 9 8 7 6 5 4 3 2 1

This work is dedicated to my Father
for His Guidance throughout my life;
to my wife Kathy
and my children:
Chris, Karoline, Keaton, and Kylie;
to my parents: Billy and Janet;
to my in-laws: Paul and Ruth;
and
to my sisters: Annette, Allison, and Amber.

Each of you has inspired me in
numerous ways, more than I can recount,
and taught me the value of love, dedication,
patience, perseverance, and caring.

REVIEWERS

Donald M. Bell, CRNA, DNSc, APN
Assistant Professor of Nurse Anesthesia
Associate Program Director for Didactic Education
College of Nursing
The University of Tennessee—Knoxville
Knoxville, Tennessee

Marjorie A. Geisz-Everson, CRNA, MS
Instructor
School of Nurse Anesthesia, Health Sciences Center
Louisiana State University
New Orleans, Louisiana

Robert M. Hovis, CRNA
Nurse Anesthetist
Department of Anesthesiology
Washington University School of Medicine
St. Louis, Missouri

Michael J. Kremer, CRNA, DNSc, FAAN
Chair, Nurse Anesthesia Department
College of Health Professions
Rosalind Franklin University of Medicine and Science
North Chicago, Illinois

Debra Pecka Malina, MS, MBA, DNSc
Certified Registered Nurse Anesthetist
Independent Contractor
Memphis, Tennessee

Daniel D. Moos, CRNA, MS
Nurse Anesthetist
Kearney Anesthesia Associates P.C.
Kearney, Nebraska
Clinical and Didactic Instructor
Bryan LGH College of Health Sciences
Lincoln, Nebraska

FOREWORD

The highest mark of professionalism is development, adoption, and utilization of standards. For decades, members of the AANA have demonstrated accountability by following standards that promote an acceptable level of patient care and criteria by which a practitioner can be measured. There are eleven standards for nurse anesthesia practice. Standard III states, "The CRNA will formulate a patient-specific plan for anesthesia care." The plan of care developed by the CRNA is based on comprehensive patient assessment, problem analysis, anticipated surgical procedure, and current anesthesia principles.

The patient with an uncommon disease is a challenge because the nurse anesthetist encounters such patients only infrequently. The goal of *Perianesthesia Patient Care for Uncommon Diseases* is to assist the anesthetist in developing an anesthesia plan by providing precise description of the pathophysiology of the diseases and aspects of their medical treatments that are relevant to the care of the patient in the perioperative period. Each of the uncommon diseases includes a section designed to relate the impact of the uncommon disease to the selection of anesthetic drugs, techniques, and monitors to be used in the perioperative period. There is liberal use of tables, boxes, and appendices to reinforce the text material. This valuable source of information is equally valuable to the beginner or the individual with experience. It serves as a quick reference for development of the anesthetic plan and is essential for busy practitioners in today's operating room environment.

The author of *Perianesthesia Patient Care for Uncommon Diseases* is an experienced clinician, teacher, mentor, and friend. We congratulate Joseph Joyce in providing the anesthesia community with a reference to guide anesthesia providers in the care of patients with unusual diseases.

Richard G. Ouellette, CRNA, M.Ed.
Sandra M. Ouellette, CRNA, M.Ed., FAAN
Past Presidents, AANA

FOREWORD

PREFACE

With each passing year we are confronted with increasingly more complex patient situations in which and for whom we are called on to provide care. The advances in physiologic and medical understanding constantly improve patients' survival. These very patients are some who, only a short time ago, would not have been able to reach an operating room to receive advanced interventions and anesthesia. Many of the patients with uncommon diseases previously would have been deemed an unacceptable anesthetic risk and, therefore would have been given very few treatment options.

This manual presents 91 uncommon diseases that may confront the perianesthesia care professional at one time or another. The emphasis of this manual is to present a brief overview of each uncommon disease: definition of the disease, incidence, disease etiology, signs and symptoms, medical management, complications, and anesthesia implications. In writing this manual my chief desire has been to give the perianesthesia care professional a starting point—a reference—for the care of a patient with an uncommon disease. This manual is here to be a rapid reference, something easy and quick to use to initially dispense with the time-consuming task of researching the particular uncommon disease; a task that could be problematic when caring for a patient requiring emergent interventions and care. My hope and desire is that this manual will help you provide the highest caliber of care to the patient with an uncommon disease and ultimately spark more curiosity on your part about a particular uncommon disease even after your obligation to one specific patient has been fulfilled.

Joseph A. Joyce, CRNA, BS

CONTENTS

Perianesthesia Patient Care *for*

UNCOMMON DISEASES

Achalasia

Definition

Achalasia is the failure to relax by the smooth muscle fibers at any junction of one part of the gastrointestinal tract with another, especially failure of the esophagogastric sphincter to relax with swallowing due to degeneration of ganglion cells in the wall of the organ.

Incidence

The incidence of achalasia is approximately 1:10,000. Patients with achalasia usually range in age from 25 to 60 years, but it may also be seen in teenagers. It is a chronic problem that worsens over time.

Etiology

The cause of achalasia is not known; the underlying problem may have a neural origin with the involvement of Auerbach's (myenteric) plexus. There are some histologic and physiologic alterations in the vagus nerve have been described in connection with the disorder.

Signs and Symptoms

- Chest pain
- Difficulty swallowing
- Heartburn
- Hiccups
- "Lump" in the throat
- Regurgitation of swallowed food, both solid and liquid
- Sense of fullness
- Weight loss

Medical Management

Achalasia is suspected based on the presence of symptoms. The following tests are performed to confirm the diagnosis: chest x-ray, barium swallow, endoscopy, and manometry.

Pharmacologic treatment is directed toward decreasing lower esophageal pressure. A calcium channel blocker or a nitrate is used most commonly to achieve this goal. The calcium

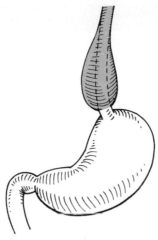

Achalasia. Decreased muscle tone and peristaltic function prevent food from entering the stomach, causing esophageal distention. (*From Phipps WP, et al: Medical-Surgical Nursing: Concepts and Clinical Practice, ed. 4, St Louis, 1991, Mosby.*)

channel blocker currently employed most often is nifedipine, while isosorbide dinitrate is the nitrate currently utilized. These medications are taken sublingually 10 to 30 minutes before meals and on an as-needed basis before bedtime if reflux is an issue during the overnight hours.

Botulinum toxin (Botox) is occasionally directly injected into the esophageal sphincter during endoscopy to restore the balance between excitatory and inhibitory neurotransmissions. Botox treatment is of limited value and duration. Treatment must be repeated in approximately 70% of patients that have been injected with Botox. Botox treatment can cause an inflammatory response in the sphincter.

The stricture can be mechanically dilated with a pneumatic (balloon) catheter. The catheter is threaded through the stricture so that the sphincter is situated at the midportion of the balloon, which is then gradually inflated to a predetermined pressure. The balloon remains inflated for a period of time after which it is deflated and the catheter withdrawn. Pneumatic dilation is successful in 70% to 80% of those treated in this manner.

Complications

- Injection of Botox can result in anaphylaxis.
- Pneumatic dilation results in esophageal perforation in approximately 5% of patients receiving this treatment. In the event of esophageal rupture or perforation, this patient is an *emergent* surgical candidate.

Anesthesia Implications

Whether treated or untreated, the patient with achalasia should receive a rapid sequence induction—a true rapid sequence induction for general anesthesia consisting of thorough preoxygenation prior to medication administration, reverse Trendelenburg's position, and respiratory "silence" after medication administration. Direct laryngoscopy and tracheal intubation should occur as quickly as possible. The patient is not a "full stomach" risk; rather, the patient should be considered a "full esophagus." "Silent" aspiration is a very real possibility in patients with achalasia.

The patient with achalasia may have had episodes of pneumonitis in the past as the result of "silent" aspiration during sleep. NPO status is *not* a guarantee that aspiration will not occur. Antacid treatment with citric acid/sodium citrate may not offer any advantage since it, too, may be stationary near the gastroesophageal junction rather than passing through the stomach.

Postoperatively the patient should be transported with oxygen by simple mask to the post-anesthesia care unit (PACU) with the head of the bed elevated ≥30 degrees to reduce the potential for reflux and aspiration of esophageal contents.

Achondroplasia (Dwarfism)

Definition

Achondroplasia is a hereditary, congenital autosomal dominant disorder that produces abnormalities in the growth and/or remodeling of cartilage and bone affecting the skull, spine, and extremities. The disorder, commonly known as dwarfism, frequently causes a person to be disproportionately short.

Incidence

The recent estimate for the incidence of achondroplasia in the United States is approximately 1:29,000; internationally, the estimate is approximately 1:40,000.

Etiology

Achondroplasia is an autosomal dominant inherited trait. The defect occurs on the short arm of chromosome 4—specifically, band 4p16.3.

Signs and Symptoms

- Abnormal odontoid
- Atlantoaxial instability
- Cleft lip
- Cleft palate
- Clubfoot
- Congenital heart disease
- Congenital odontoid absence
- Genu varum
- Hydrocephalus
- Kyphosis
- Laryngomalacia
- Micrognathia
- Obstructive sleep apnea
- Pulmonary hypertension
- Scoliosis
- Seizure disorder
- Spinal stenosis
- Tracheomalacia

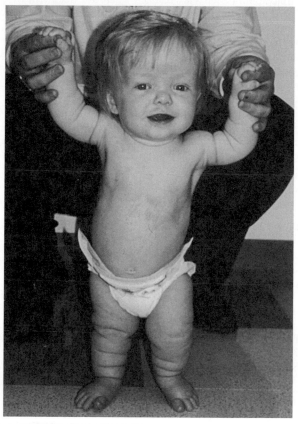

Achrondroplasia (Dwarfism). This girl has short limbs relative to trunk length. She also has a prominent forehead, low nasal root, and redundant skin folds in the arms and legs. *(From Jorde LB, et al:* Medical Genetics *[updated for 2006-2007], ed. 3, St Louis, 2006, Mosby.)*

Medical Management

The patient's short stature is frequently treated by administration of human growth hormone (somatotropin). The maximum benefits are realized when this treatment is initiated when the patient is in the age range of 1 to 6 years.

Surgical procedures may be necessary for a wide variety of occurrences, similar to any other patient. However, most procedures undertaken for patients with achondroplasia are orthopedic, with a significant portion of those involving the spine. Surgical correction of craniocervical stenosis, thoracolumbar kyphosis, spinal stenosis, lower extremities angular deformity (such as genu varum), and lengthening short extremities are frequently performed on these patients. Foramen magnum decompression and ventriculoperitoneal shunt insertion are also carried out when indicated.

Complications

- Apnea
- Brainstem compression
- Cervicomedullary compression
- Cyanosis
- Dysesthesias
- Dysphagia
- Genu varum
- Hydrocephalus
- Hypotonia
- Incontinence
- Kyphosis
- Lordosis
- Neurogenic claudication
- Obesity
- Paraparesis
- Paresthesias
- Pneumonia
- Quadriparesis
- Recurrent otitis media
- Respiratory insufficiency
- Scoliosis
- Spinal cord stenosis
- Sudden death

Anesthesia Implications

The patient with achondroplasia typically has cardiovascular and respiratory system abnormalities. Therefore the patient should have a chest x-ray, electrocardiogram, and ideally, transthoracic echocardiogram.

The patient with achondroplasia frequently has one or more craniofacial anomalies. The patient's airway must be thoroughly assessed preoperatively. The anesthetist should prepare for encountering a difficult airway. The patient with achondroplasia frequently has laryngomalacia and subglottic stenosis; thus a smaller than "calculated" endotracheal tube should be within easy reach. The urgent need to surgically secure this patient's airway should be anticipated.

Another possible impediment to securing the patient's airway is an extremely limited range of motion of the neck as the result of atlantoaxial instability. The patient's range of motion should be observed preoperatively and prominently documented before surgery and anesthesia. The anesthetist must not attempt to hyperextend the patient's neck because the atlantoaxial joint may be easily dislocated with high compromise of the spinal cord, possibly resulting in quadriplegia.

Pulmonary volumes may be altered significantly by kyphosis. The patient's respiratory function should be evaluated extensively preoperatively via chest x-ray, arterial blood gas analysis, and pulmonary function testing.

Laryngeal mask airways (LMAs) may be utilized on the patient with achondroplasia. The use of such an airway device should be appropriate for the proposed surgical intervention and may facilitate tracheal intubation in a difficult situation.

Because of associated restrictive pulmonary disease, higher respiratory rates with reduced ventilatory volume may be required. This may be associated with high ventilatory pressures. As a result, pressure-controlled ventilation methods may provide better respiratory exchange and reduce the risk of air trapping and barotrauma.

Regional anesthesia is acceptable for the patient with achondroplasia, but the patient's degree of kyphoscoliosis may make instillation difficult. The anesthetist must be aware that even a relatively small volume of anesthetic may spread more than expected and cause a higher subarachnoid block than originally intended.

Positioning is critical particularly because of the patient's atlantoaxial joint instability. The patient's head and neck must be maintained in a neutral position at all times. Movement of the patient must be slow and deliberate, especially when the patient must be placed in either the lateral decubitus or the prone position.

Postoperative pain control may be a challenge. The patient with achondroplasia may have obstructive sleep apnea, and the effects of opioid analgesics on the respiratory system may be magnified by the obstructive tendencies.

Acromegaly

Definition

Acromegaly is the abnormal enlargement of limbs and facial features as a result of hypersecretion of growth hormone after maturity. The disease is usually the result of a pituitary tumor.

Incidence

The incidence of acromegaly is estimated to be 3:1,000,000 to 4:1,000,000.

Etiology

More than 95% of growth hormone–releasing hormone (GHRH) independent cases of acromegaly are the result of growth hormone (GH)–secreting pituitary adenoma. These adenomas are either macroadenomas (>1 cm) or microadenomas (<1 cm). Macroadenomas predominate, accounting for more than 80% of the tumors.

Signs and Symptoms

- Arthritis
- Bitemporal hemianopia
- Congestive heart failure
- Enlarged thyroid
- Enlarging extremities
- Facial feature coarsening
- Frontal bossing
- Headaches
- Hypercalciuria
- Hyperhidrosis
- Hyperphosphatemia
- Hypertriglyceridemia
- Increased incidence of CHF
- Increased incidence of colonic polyps
- Increased incidence of glucose intolerance
- Increased obstructive apnea
- Increased shoe or ring size

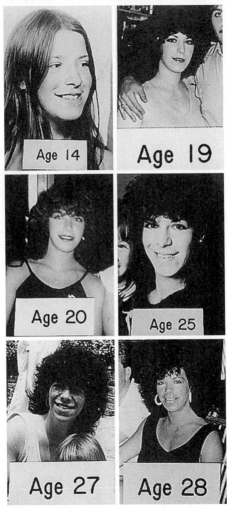

Acromegaly. Chronologic sequence of photographs showing slow development of acromegaly. (*From Belchetz P, Hammond P*: Mosby's Color Atlas and Text of Diabetes and Endocrinology, *Edinburgh, 2003, Mosby.*)

- Macroglossia
- Mild hirsutism (females)
- Multinodular goiter
- Nose thickening
- Prognathism
- Soft tissue swelling

Medical Management

The goal of treatment for acromegaly is symptom alleviation via a multimodal treatment plan. The *first* line of treatment is surgical removal of the pituitary tumor, which is 80% to 85% successful for microadenomas and 50% to 65% successful for macroadenomas. When complete remission is not achieved by surgical excision of the tumor, somatostatin analogues, dopamine analogues, and growth hormone receptor antagonists dominate subsequent medical management.

Complications

If left untreated, acromegaly produces somatic hypertrophy in all organ systems, including the heart muscle, soft tissue, and kidneys. Articular overgrowth of synovial tissue and hypertrophic arthropathy cause joint and back pain. Soft tissue overgrowth also produces thick skin, hyperhidrosis (malodorous), and carpal tunnel syndrome. Macroglossia can produce obstructive sleep apnea.

Hypertrophic growth of the heart produces hypertension, left ventricular hypertrophy, and acromegalic cardiomyopathy with dysfunction and dysrhythmias.

Anesthesia Implications

Soft tissue thickening may increase the challenge of obtaining intravenous access.

Hypertrophy of the tongue and mandible may interfere with securing an adequate mask fit during induction of anesthesia. Direct visualization of the glottis may also be more difficult. A difficult airway cart with fiberoptic capabilities should be on hand when caring for the patient with acromegaly. Surgical tracheostomy may be required if intubation becomes impossible.

The patient may have mild diabetes mellitus, ventricular hypertrophy, hypertension, degenerative vascular disease, and cardiac disease. Intraoperative monitoring of capillary blood glucose levels with or without insulin coverage may therefore be appropriate.

The patient may be more susceptible to cardiac ischemia.

Venous air embolism is a real concern during transsphenoidal surgery.

Steroid coverage and prophylactic antibiotics should be administered.

Because of the patient's propensity toward obstructive sleep apnea, short-acting medications, whether inhalational or intravenous, should dominate the anesthetic plan. Sevoflurane, propofol, and remifentanil are all appropriate choices to allow for relatively rapid change in the depth of anesthesia, along with rapid induction and emergence.

Muscle paralysis must be fully reversed to minimize recurization phenomenon and airway obstruction.

Extubation should not occur until the patient has good control of the airway reflexes; however, the anesthetist must take care that the patient not dislodge the nasal packing in place as a result of the transsphenoidal tumor resection.

Throat packing must be removed before extubation. Although this may seem a trivial, common sense matter, this simple step has been overlooked in the past and has been the cause of serious airway emergencies.

Narcotic administration, intraoperatively and postoperatively, must be done with caution because of the potential of sleep apnea.

For the patient with sleep apnea, nasal continuous positive airway pressure (CPAP) will not be an option, particularly if the transsphenoidal approach has been used.

Acute Leukemia

Definition

Leukemia is a progressive, malignant disease of the blood-forming tissues marked by a distorted proliferation and development of leukocytes and their precursors in the blood and bone marrow.

Acute leukemia is a subtype in which the involved cell line shows little or no differentiation and usually consists of blast cells. This subtype is further differentiated into *acute myelogenous leukemia* (AML) and *acute lymphocytic/lymphoblastic leukemia* (ALL).

Incidence

The incidence of AML is approximately 4:100,000. It is the more common form of acute leukemia, accounting for about 80% of diagnosed adult cases. Acute leukemia is more common in Caucasians and in males. It accounts for about 20% of cases of childhood leukemia.

ALL, the most common form of malignancy in childhood, makes up approximately 33% of all pediatric cancers. It also occurs more frequently in Caucasians. Overall, the incidence is about 30:1,000,000. For children younger than 15 years of age, the incidence of ALL in Caucasians is about 33:1,000,000, and in African Americans it is about 15:1,000,000. The disease accounts for about 80% of cases of childhood leukemia.

Etiology

Acute leukemia is not fully understood but is believed to have multiple causes. Several factors have been identified as increasing the risk for developing acute leukemia, including bone marrow damage, retroviruses, and genetic disorders such as Klinefelter syndrome or Down syndrome.

Signs and Symptoms

- Bleeding
- Bone pain
- Cranial nerve involvement (third, fourth, sixth, and seventh cranial nerves)
- Dyspnea
- Fatigue
- Fever
- Headache
- Hepatosplenomegaly
- Irritability
- Lethargy
- Lymphadenopathy
- Nausea and vomiting
- Nuchal rigidity
- Pallor
- Papilledema
- Petechiae
- Signs of bone marrow failure (e.g., anemia, thrombocytopenia, neutropenia)
- Weight loss

Medical Management

AML

Chemotherapy is the first line of treatment for AML, although only a minority of patients are cured.

Treatment is typically with an anthracycline drug singly or with an anthracenedione drug combined with arabinosyl cytosine.

Transfusion with packed cells should be administered when the patient's hemoglobin concentration is less than 7 to 8 g/dL, or at a higher concentration in the event of cardiovascular or pulmonary compromise.

Platelets should be transfused when the count is below 10,000 to 20,000/μL. In cases of pulmonary or gastrointestinal bleeding, transfuse platelets even if the count is more than 50,000/μL; and in cases of cerebral hemorrhage, when the count is more than 100,000/μL.

Fresh frozen plasma is administered when there is a significantly prolonged physical therapy (PT).

Cryoprecipitate is given when the patient's fibrinogen concentration is less than 100 g/dL.

The patient who becomes febrile should receive an antibiotic, which should be a third-generation cephalosporin and may or may not be combined with vancomycin.

If the patient remains febrile despite 3 to 5 days of antibiotic therapy, antifungal agents should be administered.

ALL

ALL is treated primarily with chemotherapy. For a pediatric patient, the chemotherapy agents must be administered via a centrally located, indwelling catheter or well.

Complications

Mortality is typically the consequence of pancytopenia, infection, hemorrhage, renal dysfunction, or hepatic dysfunction. Uric acid nephropathy is common in a patient with leukemia. Uric acid is produced faster than the kidneys can clear it and, as a result, precipitates in the renal tubules, culminating in renal failure.

Anesthesia Implications

Anemia decreases the oxygenation of tissues both as a result of decreased carrying capacity and a "left shift" in the O_2 dissociation curve. The reduced oxygen delivery ability results in the need for increased heart rate and thus higher myocardial oxygen consumption and demand.

Thrombocytopenia can contribute to preoperative blood loss from gastrointestinal bleeding or from hemoptysis, resulting in decreased intravascular volume. Transfusion of packed cells, platelets, fresh frozen plasma, and/or cryoprecipitate may be necessary before surgery and anesthesia. Vasodilation from general anesthesia induction or instillation of a regional anesthetic can produce profound hypotension. The patient with leukemia should be adequately hydrated before initiation of an anesthetic plan.

Acute Porphyria

Definition

Porphyria, in general, is a broad disease category that encompasses eight distinct, related disorders. The acute variants may be characterized by demonstration of abdominal pain, neuropathy, autonomic instability, and/or psychosis.

Acute Porphyria and Enzyme Deficiency		
Acute Variant	Heme Pathway Intermediary	Deficient Enzyme
Plumboporphyria	Gamma-aminolevulinic acid (γ-ALA)	ALA dehydratase
Acute intermittent	Porphobilinogen (PBG)	PBG deaminase
Hereditary Porphyria		
Coproporphyria	Coproporphyrinogen	Coproporphyrinogen oxidase
Variegate porphyria	Protoporphyrinogen	Protoporphyrinogen oxidase

Incidence

The estimated incidence of acute porphyria is variable. Across Europe, the overall incidence is about 1:20,000; in northern Sweden, the incidence is about 1:10,000. Internationally, the estimated incidence is about 5:100,000.

Etiology

Each acute porphyria variant is produced by an inherited deficiency of a specific enzyme required for progression through the pathway to completion of heme production.

Signs and Symptoms

- Abdominal pain
- Agitation
- Anxiety
- Aphasia
- Apraxia
- Bladder dysfunction
- Confusion
- Cortical blindness
- Depression
- Dysesthesias
- Dysuria
- Encephalopathy
- Fever
- Guillain-Barré–like syndrome
- Hallucinations
- Hyperhidrosis
- Hypersecretion of catecholamines
- Hypertension
- Insomnia
- Mild-to-severe paresthesias
- Motor nerve palsies (especially cranial nerves VII and X)
- Nausea
- Numbness
- Optic nerve dysfunction (may deteriorate to blindness)
- Paranoia
- Partial ileus
- Rhabdomyolysis
- Seizures
- Tachycardia
- Tremor
- Urine color changes to red or becomes very dark when exposed to light
- Vomiting

Medical Management

For the patient with an acute porphyria variant, the first-line intervention during an acute episode begins with removal of any initiating medication or agent. The patient should receive intravenous hydration with carbohydrate-containing solutions, such as dextrose 10%. Abdominal pain should be controlled with opioid analgesics; nausea and vomiting that occurs should be treated with phenothiazine agents. Should these interventions fail to provide symptomatic relief, an intravenous infusion of heme is generally initiated for a period ranging from 3 to 14 days.

If the patient with an acute porphyria experiences seizures, the first intervention should be to determine serum electrolyte concentrations and serum osmolarity as quickly as possible. Acute porphyria patients are prone to develop hyponatremia as well as syndrome of inappropriate antidiuretic hormone (SIADH), either of which can result in seizure. Immediate control of seizures can be achieved with intravenous diazepam or magnesium sulfate to allow time for laboratory tests to be

completed and the results transmitted. Correction of electrolyte imbalances may reverse the seizures. If epilepsy is the
concurrent cause, seizure control can be safely attained with
gabapentin. Rectal administration of diazepam may be necessary to achieve a useful degree of seizure control.

Autonomic instability that may accompany an acute episode
can be successfully managed using β-blocking agents. Acute
hypertension should be treated quickly to prevent development of undesirable sequelae, such as stroke. Phenothiazine
medications, effective against episodes of nausea and vomiting,
also help control any psychiatric symptoms that may arise.

Complications

- Adrenergic crisis
- Chronic renal insufficiency
- Hypertension
- Paralysis
- Seizures

Anesthesia Implications

One of the first decisions the anesthetist must make when
caring for the patient with an acute porphyria is which drugs
may be safely used. Many drugs used by the anesthetist are
known or suspected to precipitate an acute episode.

Drugs Known to Precipitate an Acute Porphyria Attack	
• Alcohol	• Methohexital (Brevital)
• Amphetamines	• Nifedipine (Adalat, Procardia)
• Carbamazepine	• Pentazocine (Talwin)
• Carisoprodol (Soma, Vanadom)	• Phenacetin
• Clonazepam (Klonopin)	• Phenytoin (Dilantin)
• Cocaine	• Primidone (Mysoline)
• Danazol (Danocrine)	• Progesterone
• Diclofenac	• Pyrazinamide
• Ecstasy (MDMA)	• Pyrazolones
• Ergots	• Rifampin (Rifadin, Rimactane)
• Estrogens	• Synthetic progestins
• Etomidate (Amidate)	• Thiamylal (Surital)
• Ketorolac (Acular, Toradol)	• Thiopental (Pentothal)
• Marijuana	

Factors that Provoke an Acute Porphyria Attack

- Alcohol ingestion or abuse
- Cigarette smoking
- Endogenous hormones
- Extreme dieting/fasting/low-to-zero carbohydrate diet
- Infection
- Menstruation
- Psychological stress
- Surgery

Drugs Available to Use in Patients with Acute Porphyria

Nonprecipitating
- Acetaminophen
- Alfentanil (Alfenta)
- α Agonists
- Aspirin
- Atropine (Atro-Pen, Sal-Tropine)
- β Agonists
- β Antagonists
- Bupivacaine
- Codeine
- Droperidol (Inapsine)
- Epinephrine
- Erythromycin
- Fentanyl
- Gabapentin (Neurontin)
- Glucocorticoids
- Glycopyrrolate (Robinul)
- Insulin
- Lidocaine (Xylocaine)
- Mepivacaine
- Morphine
- Naloxone (Narcan)
- Neostigmine (Prostigmin)
- Nitrous oxide
- Pancuronium (Pavulon)
- Propofol (Diprivan, disoprofol [Disphrol])
- Ropivacaine (Naropin)
- Succinylcholine (Anectine)
- Sufentanil (Sufenta)
- Tetracaine (Pontocaine)

Possibly Nonprecipitating
- Atracurium (Tracrium)
- Cimetidine (Tagamet)
- Cisatracurium (Nimbex)
- Desflurane (Suprane)
- Diltiazem
- Isoflurane (Forane)
- Ketamine (Ketalar)
- Lorazepam (Ativan)
- Metoclopramide
- Midazolam (Versed)
- Mivacurium (Mivacron)
- Nitroprusside (Nitropress)
- Ondansetron (Zofran)
- Ranitidine (Zantac)
- Rocuronium (Zemuron)
- Sevoflurane (Ultane)
- Vecuronium (Norcuron)

Preoperatively the anesthetist must focus on several aspects of the patient's condition. Fluid and electrolyte balance should be well documented before surgery and anesthesia. An imbalance of either should be corrected before anesthesia is initiated. Hyponatremia is frequently associated with development of seizures. The patient's muscle strength and cranial nerve function must be assessed. Both may affect the patient's ability to maintain respiratory function postoperatively without artificial assistance.

On the day of the operation, the patient with acute porphyria should have fluid and caloric intake restrictions shortened to the least amount of time considered safe to provide anesthesia. Prolonged restrictions may trigger an acute attack. The impact of the necessary restrictions may be eased somewhat by infusing glucose-containing, electrolyte-balanced solutions after securing intravenous access. The patient must also receive an anxiolytic premedication to reduce anxiety and stress, which can also precipitate an acute attack.

General anesthesia can be safely administered to the patient with an acute porphyria; however, this technique does significantly increase the potential of an acute attack. Both propofol and ketamine have been used without incident in patients with acute porphyria. Once general anesthesia is induced, the patient can be maintained using any of the volatile inhalational agents currently available. Regional anesthesia is also a safe, viable technique for the patient with acute porphyria. Each of the available local anesthetics, such as lidocaine and mepivacaine, has been used without negative effects with regard to the patient's porphyria. However, there are contraindications to regional anesthesia, including unstable hemodynamics, reduced mental capacity, and/or confusion.

The anesthetist must be alert for signs and symptoms of an acute porphyria attack. These can be subtle in the patient who is already receiving general anesthesia. The anesthetist must watch for the sudden appearance of tachycardia and hypertension that may be inappropriate to the degree of surgical stimulation and that are minimally responsive to administration of an opioid analgesic and/or increased volatile inhalational agent. In such circumstances, initial treatment may be administration of a β-adrenergic blocking agent. The anesthetist may confirm the suspicion of an acute attack by testing for increased levels of porphobilinogen (PBG).

During an acute attack, urinary PBG may be 20 to 200 mg/mL. Trace PBG kits are commercially available that can detect levels of ≥6 mg/L to confirm the suspicion. The anesthetist must simultaneously initiate measures to ensure adequate hydration and provide some carbohydrate intravenously. It would be prudent to add a dextrose-containing solution to an existing intravenous line or start a dedicated line.

Prevention of nausea and/or vomiting should be undertaken as well. The anesthetist should insert a nasogastric tube to evacuate the stomach contents and keep it empty. This symptomatic pain should be attacked pharmacologically by administration of a phenothiazine agent or ondansetron for the patient who is particularly sensitive to the extrapyramidal effects of phenothiazines. If a seizure ensues, particularly in a patient with a regional anesthetic, diazepam is quite useful in interrupting the seizure activity. On confirmation of an acute attack, the anesthetist should initiate treatment with the single available treatment medication, hemin (in the United States). Hemin corrects the heme deficiency and suppresses the concentration of porphyrin precursors. The dosage is 1 to 4 mg/kg/day and should be infused over 10 to 15 minutes. The dose may be repeated no more frequently than every 12 hours and the maximum daily dose cannot exceed 6 mg/kg/day. This treatment regimen should be continued for 3 to 14 days.

Ankylosing Spondylosis

Definition

Ankylosing spondylosis (AS) is rheumatoid arthritis of the spine found predominately in persons 20 to 40 years of age. It produces pain and stiffness as a result of inflammation of the sacroiliac, intervertebral, and costovertebral joints. The AS disease process may progress to complete spinal and thoracic rigidity.

Incidence

In the United States, the incidence of AS is approximately 0.1% to 0.2% of the population. Internationally, it accounts for 0.1% to 1.0% of the population. In persons with the HLA-B27 antigen, the incidence is 1% to 2%.

Etiology

The cause of AS is not fully understood. There seems to be a strong genetic predisposition, specifically involving human leukocyte antigen (HLA). HLA-B27 is believed to resemble and/or act as a receptor for a causative antigen (e.g., a type of bacteria). Currently, spurious evidence points to a bacterial causative agent, such as *Klebsiella pneumoniae*.

Signs and Symptoms

- Age younger than 40 years (usually)
- Chest tightness
- Decreased range of motion of costovertebral and costotransverse joints
- Difficulty breathing
- Elevated alkaline phosphatase
- Elevated C-reactive protein
- Elevated creatinine kinase
- Elevated erythrocyte sedimentation rate
- Fever
- Insidious onset of low back pain, with exacerbations and remissions
- Morning stiffness
- Pain and/or swelling of insertions of ligaments and tendons

- Peripheral enthesitis
- Stooped forward, flexed head/neck position due to cervical and upper spine fusion
- Temporomandibular joint pain and decreased range of motion
- Weight loss

Medical Management

Preventive or prophylactic measures for AS are not available. AS is not surgically preventable, although surgical intervention may repair complications that occur as a result of the disease. The pain and inflammation of the joints are generally treated pharmacologically with nonsteroidal anti-inflammatory drugs

Ossification of disks, joints, and ligaments of spinal column

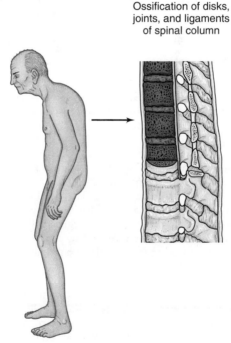

Ankylosing Spondylosis. Characteristic posture and primary pathologic sites of inflammation and resulting damage. *(From McCance KL, Huether SE:* Pathophysiology: The Biologic Basis for Disease in Adults and Children, *ed. 5, St Louis, 2006, Mosby.)*

(NSAIDs). Sulfasalazine is used as an adjunct medication with reported effectiveness for patients with peripheral joint involvement and/or concomitant inflammatory bowel disease. Sulfasalazine is generally reserved for the patient who is unresponsive to NSAIDs or for whom NSAIDs are contraindicated. Methotrexate is typically the tertiary pharmacologic therapy for the patient with pain and symptoms inadequately controlled by NSAIDs and/or sulfasalazine.

Complications

- Atlantoaxial subluxation
- Death
- Gastrointestinal bleeding
- Inflammatory bowel disease
- Limited functional ability
- Pain
- Spinal cord compression
- Stiffness
- Ulceration of gastrointestinal mucosa
- Vertebral fractures

Anesthesia Implications

The most frequently affected vertebrae are those in the cervical spine. Atlantoaxial subluxation is a very real and serious potential problem for the anesthetist to encounter. The patient typically presents with significantly to severely limited range of motion (ROM) of the cervical vertebrae (neck). In addition, the temporomandibular joint may have a very limited ROM, resulting in a restricted ability to open the mouth. These factors may make direct laryngoscopy difficult or completely impossible. A laryngeal mask airway (LMA) may be an appropriate tool for securing the patient's airway, depending on the proposed surgical procedure. In some cases, an LMA may be required to achieve tracheal intubation. The anesthetist must also be prepared to perform an awake fiberoptic intubation.

As a result of the fusion of the costovertebral joint, the chest wall may be permanently fixed in what appears to be an inspiratory position. Chest wall compliance is dramatically reduced and the functional residual capacity (FRC) is increased. These changes place considerably more importance on the diaphragm for the breathing cycle. The loss of chest wall compliance minimizes the contributions of the accessory muscles, particularly the intercostal muscles, for inspiration and expiration. Therefore any intrusion on diaphragmatic excursion seriously compromises the respiratory cycle of the patient with AS. For example, thoracic or extensive abdominal surgical procedures increase the stress placed on the diaphragm and, as a result, it may be necessary to provide prolonged ventilatory support. The expiratory phase of the ventilatory cycle should be longer than normal to reduce the possibility of lung hyperinflation.

Placement of spinal or epidural needles may be difficult or even impossible because of the ossification of the interspinous ligaments along with the development of bony ridges between the vertebrae (syndesmophytes).

Extreme care must be taken during patient positioning, even in the supine position. Spinal rigidity and osteoporosis significantly limit the degree of flexibility the patient has and the degree of movement that can be tolerated before significant spinal injury will be incurred. Even in the supine position, extra cervical support in the form of pillows or blankets may be required for the patient's comfort. Placing the patient in either the lateral decubitus or the prone position makes it imperative that the anesthetist be more cautious, gentle, and deliberate in maintaining the head and neck in as nearly neutral a position as possible to avoid even minor trauma and the possibility of a devastating spinal injury.

Arnold-Chiari Malformation

Definition

Arnold-Chiari malformation is a complex congenital malformation of the hindbrain that is often associated with myelomeningocele. The deformity is characterized by downward
displacement of the medulla, fourth ventricle, and cerebellum
into the spinal canal. The pons and fourth ventricle are elon-
gated, which is believed to be the result of the relatively small
posterior fossa. It is the most common, serious malformation
of the posterior fossa. Arnold-Chiari is also known as Chiari II
malformation (CM II).

Incidence

Recent estimates are that the frequency of this malformation in
the United States is approximately 1:1000.

Etiology

This congenital anomaly is a complex entity that involves the
skull, dura, brain, spine, and spinal cord. The association with
myelomeningocele is almost 100%. Several theories have been
advocated to explain the development of the Arnold-Chiari
malformation.

The various theories can be classed into two schools of
thought. The first ascribes the malformation to mechanical
factors, and the second finds the cause to be abnormal
embryologic development. The "mechanical forces school" uses
theories of hydrodynamics and traction. The "embryologic
school" includes theories on developmental arrest, primary
dysgenesis, small posterior fossa, hindbrain overgrowth,
neuroschisis, and neurulation abnormalities. One of the simpler
and widely accepted theories suggests that the condition arises
when a cerebellum of normal size or proportion develops in
a posterior fossa that is abnormally small with a low tentorial
attachment.

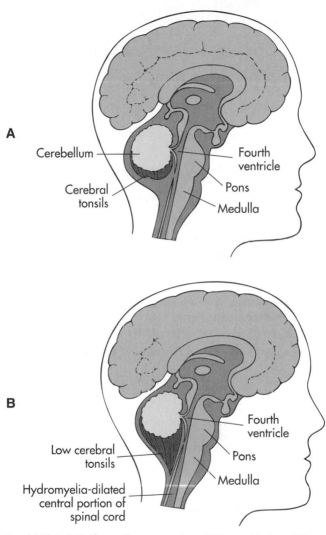

Arnold-Chiari Malformation. Comparison of **(A)** normal brain and **(B)** Arnold-Chiari type II malformation. *(From McCance KL, Huether SE:* Patho–physiology: The Biologic Basis for Disease in Adults and Children, *ed. 5, St Louis, 2006, Mosby.)*

Signs and Symptoms

Infancy
- Aspiration
- Bladder and/or bowel function degradation
- Depressed/absent gag reflex
- Episodic apnea
- Fixed retrocollis
- Impaired swallowing
- Nystagmus
- Respiratory distress
- Scoliosis
- Upper and lower extremities pain
- Weak/absent cry

Childhood
- Appendicular and/or truncal ataxia
- Depressed/absent cough reflex
- Exaggerated deep tendon reflexes
- Gastroesophageal reflux
- Gradual function loss
- Mirror movements
- Nystagmus (horizontal and rotatory)
- Recurrent pneumonia secondary to aspiration
- Spastic quadriparesis
- Syncopal episodes
- Upper extremity weakness with increased tone

Medical Management

Medical management of the patient with Arnold-Chiari malformation primarily involves surgical interventions. Hydrocephalus develops in about 80% of patients with Arnold-Chiari malformation, and they often present as a medical emergency in need of insertion of a shunt for relief of the intracranial pressure. In addition to hydrocephalus, the patient may have several associated abnormalities and may require general anesthesia to facilitate the corrective surgical intervention(s).

Complications

- Brainstem dysfunction
- Cranial nerve dysfunction
- Mortality: 10% to 15% in the first 2 years; some report long-term rates of up to 50%
- Respiratory difficulties (apnea, inspiratory stridor, prolonged expiratory apnea with cyanosis [PEAC])

Anomalies Associated with Arnold-Chiari Malformation

- Aqueductal stenosis
- Contracted narrow gyria
- Corpus callosium dysgenesis
- Diastematomyelia
- Heterotopias
- Low-lying, often-tethered conus medullaris below the L_2 nerve
- Malrotation of C_1 and C_2 arches
- Myelomeningocele
- Obstructive hydrocephalus
- Segmented anomalies/incomplete C_1 arch
- Septum pellucidum absence
- Syringohydromyelia

Rare Anomalies
- Cervical myelocystocele
- Frontometaphyseal dysplasia
- Holoprosencephaly
- Juvenile distal spinal muscular dystrophy
- Williams syndrome (see p. 351)

Anesthesia Implications

The associated myelomeningocele is generally surgically corrected within the first hours of the neonate's life. This intervention frequently employs local anesthetic infiltration or general anesthesia. The primary objective is to close the defect to minimize the potential for central nervous system infection. Awake intubation of the neonate while in the lateral decubitus position is elected to avoid compression of the meningocele sac. The neonate may be placed in the supine position, so long as the meningocele sac is "insulated" from direct pressure by elevating the child's body with a foam ring, or "doughnut." Anesthesia can be maintained with volatile inhalational agents with mechanical ventilation. Functional neural elements have to be assessed by the surgeon; therefore, long-acting muscle relaxants should not be used. The patient is maintained in the prone position postoperatively. If the patient is extubated, respiratory status should be assessed constantly. The patient with Arnold-Chiari malformation has abnormal responses to hypoxia and hypercarbia and is also at increased risk for aspiration because of higher incidences of gastroesophageal reflux and abnormal vocal cord mobility. Finally, the patient with a myelomeningocele has a substantially higher incidence of latex sensitivity and/or true allergy; therefore it is prudent to take latex precautions.

The most common surgical intervention for the patient with Arnold-Chiari malformation is exploration of the posterior fossa. Other surgical interventions employed include suboccipital craniectomy, C_1/C_2 laminectomy, subarachnoid adhesions lysis, dural band incision, and duraplasty. Preoperatively, the patient's neural function must be assessed with particular attention to upper airway control, protection from aspiration, and gas exchange. The appearance or exacerbation of neural symptoms during neck flexion and extension must be determined. The patient must also be assessed for the presence or absence of increased intracranial pressure (ICP).

The neck should be placed in an anatomic alignment as neutral as possible, and great care should be taken to avoid extremes in flexion or extension to avoid potential compression of neural structures. Increased ICP is always a potential development even with a shunt in place, and the anesthesia should be administered with this in mind. Mild hyperventilation to reduce the Pa_{CO_2} will help thwart the development of increased ICP. The anesthetist must also be prepared for potentially large volumes of blood loss if the transverse and/or torcular sinuses should be violated. When the patient is in the semi-sitting or prone positions, air embolism is a very real threat.

Arthrogryposis

Definition

Arthrogryposis is a nonprogressive condition that is obvious at birth by the characteristic multiple joint contractures that occur throughout the body. The disorder is also known as arthrogryposis multiplex congenita.

Incidence

The incidence of arthrogryposis is about 1:3000 live births without racial or gender preference.

Causes of Fetal Akinesia	
• Attempted pregnancy termination • Carbon monoxide poisoning or severe hypoxia during pregnancy • Chronic amniotic fluid leak • Demise of a twin • Infants of mothers with myotonic dystrophy, myasthenia gravis, multiple sclerosis • Large uterine fibroids or tumors • Maternal fever >39° C (>102.2° F) for an extended time	• Maternal hyperthermia • Maternal infections (rubella, rubeola, coxsackievirus, enterovirus, or Akabane) • Multiple fetuses • Oligohydramnios • Severe hypotension at a critical time • Teratogens (drugs, alcohol, curare, methocarbamol, phenytoin)

Etiology

The underlying cause of arthrogryposis is fetal akinesia. Fetal abnormalities—such as neurogenic, muscular or connective tissue disorders, limitations to mechanical movement—or maternal disorders—such as infections, substance abuse, trauma, or maternal illness—may be the cause of fetal akinesia. Fetal akinesia results in development of excess connective tissue around the joint. The joint becomes fixed and the limited movement within the uterus further exacerbates the joint contracture.

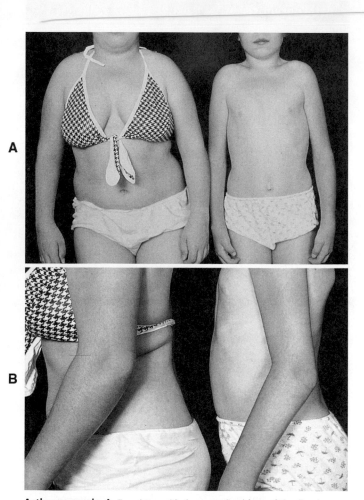

Arthrogryposis. A, Two sisters with the generalized form of the disorder. Note the stiff posture and tubular appearance of the limbs. Motion of all joints is limited as a result of failure in the development of or degeneration of muscular structures. Their stature is short. **B,** The lateral view highlights the flexion of contractures of the elbows. *(From Zitelli BJ, Davis HW: Atlas of Pediatric Physical Diagnosis, ed. 5, St. Louis, 2007, Mosby.)*

Syndromes Associated with Arthrogryposis	
• Bowen-Conradi syndrome*	• Mietens syndrome*
• C syndrome (Opitz trigonocephaly syndrome)*	• Miller-Dieker syndrome
• Faciocardiomelic syndrome*	• Syndrome of cloudy cornea/ diaphragmatic defect/distal limb deformities
• Fetal alcohol syndrome	
• FG syndrome*	• Toriello-Bauserman syndrome*
• Marden-Walker syndrome*	• Zellweger syndrome*
• Meckel syndrome*	

*See Appendix G: Rare Syndromes.

Signs and Symptoms

- Absence of muscles or muscle groups
- Absent patella
- Aortic stenosis
- Cleft palate
- Coarctation of the aorta
- Craniosynostosis
- Cryptorchidism
- Cutis marmorata
- Cyanotic heart disease
- Dislocated radial heads
- Distally increasing severity of deformity
- Facial asymmetry
- Flat nasal bridge
- Fusiform or cylindrical shape of involved extremities
- Hemangioma
- Hypertelorism
- Hypoplastic diaphragm
- Inguinal/umbilical hernia
- Joint dislocations
- Joint rigidity
- Lack of labia
- Limb shortening
- Limited jaw range of motion
- Microencephaly
- Micrognathism
- Microphallus
- Muscle atrophy
- Pterygia across joints
- Ptosis
- Pulmonary hypoplasia
- Renal anomalies
- Scoliosis
- Strabismus
- Symmetric deformities
- Tracheal and/or laryngeal clefts or stenosis
- Trismus

Medical Management

Medical management of arthrogryposis consists primarily of physical therapy. The goal is to attain and maintain limb alignment and establish joint stability so the patient will eventually be able to ambulate. Gentle manipulation and stretching result in improved range of motion. Best results are obtained when therapy is initiated soon after birth. Late manipulation is not very productive. Casting for immobility is somewhat counterproductive. Splinting overnight is preferred in combination with physical therapy.

The patient who has severe trismus may require feeding assistance, such as a feeding gastrostomy or nasogastric feeding tube. The patient may require intubation or tracheostomy for respiratory support.

Surgical intervention is sometimes required. At an early age, such as 3 to 12 months, a single-stage bone and tendon transfer procedure should be undertaken. More intricate procedures, such as opponensplasty, may be contemplated at later developmental/growth stages to improve function. Generally, soft tissue procedures are performed at an early age; osteotomies are performed only after growth is completed. Specific joints are generally addressed individually.

Complications

- Craniofacial deformities
- Fractures
- Osseous hypoplasia
- Scoliosis

Anesthesia Implications

The patient who requires feeding assistance may be chronically dehydrated and may have electrolyte imbalances. Similar to a patient with muscular diseases, the patient with arthrogryposis may experience heightened sensitivity or other altered responses to muscle relaxants, both depolarizing and nondepolarizing.

Of particular importance is the association of malignant hyperthermia in the patient who has a form of arthrogryposis with multiple pterygium syndrome.

Vascular access may be difficult to obtain in part because of the joint contractures.

Thorough cardiac assessment should be completed preoperatively. The patient with arthrogryposis is prone to cardiac anomalies, including aortic stenosis, coarctation of the aorta, and cyanotic heart disease.

The patient with arthrogryposis may have craniofacial anomalies such as micrognathia or high-arched palate as well as cervical spine abnormalities. As a result, securing the patient's airway may prove difficult and may be deemed impossible. The fiberoptic bronchoscope, intubating laryngeal mask airway, and other difficult airway equipment should be immediately on hand. If these measures prove unsuccessful, a tracheostomy may be required. In addition, the patient's normal respiratory function may be a very precarious balance because of associated malformations such as tracheal and laryngeal clefts, and/or stenosis, weak muscles, hypoplasia, or hypoplastic diaphragm. Therefore the anesthetist should anticipate the need for postoperative ventilatory support.

The multiple joint contractures may make it difficult to position the patient. Positioning must also be undertaken with care and caution to minimize the risk of fractures.

Autonomic Hyperreflexia

Definition

Autonomic hyperreflexia is an imbalanced reflex sympathetic discharge that occurs in patients with spinal cord injury (SCI) higher than the level of splanchnic sympathetic outflow. Autonomic hyperreflexia is also known as autonomic dysreflexia (AD).

Incidence

Approximately 65% to 85% of patients with SCI above the T_7 level experience autonomic hyperreflexia. Prevalence rates vary, with the incidence occurring in 48% to 90% of the patients with an injury above T_6. Because the male to female ratio of SCI is 4:1, that same ratio applies to the incidence of autonomic hyperreflexia.

Etiology

Autonomic hyperreflexia is typically seen after the post-injury period of spinal shock has "run its course" and some reflexes have returned. These intact peripheral sensory nerves transmit to the spinothalamic and posterior columns, which then return impulses via the sympathetic neurons located in the intermediolateral gray matter. The inhibitory mechanisms above the SCI are not transmittable past the level of the SCI; thus the sympathetic stimulation is unopposed and can produce serious vasoconstriction, bradycardia, and other symptoms. The box on p. 37 lists stimuli that produce or trigger an episode of autonomic hyperreflexia.

Signs and Symptoms

- Bradycardia
- Cardiac dysrhythmias
- Cerebral hemorrhage
- Convulsions
- Erythematous rash
- Headache
- Hypertension
- Nasal congestion
- Piloerection below the level of the lesion

- Profuse sweating
- Pulmonary edema
- Vasoconstriction below the lesion level

- Vasodilation above the lesion level
- Vision changes

Stimuli/Triggers of Autonomic Hyperreflexia

- Abdominal pathology/trauma
- Appendicitis
- Bladder distention
- Blister
- Burns/sunburn
- Constrictive clothes, shoes, appliances
- Contact with hard or sharp objects
- Cystoscopy
- Deep vein thrombosis
- Detrusor-sphincter dyssynergia
- Ejaculation
- Epididymitis
- Fractures
- Gallstones
- Gastric ulcers
- Gastritis
- Gastrocolic irritation
- Hemorrhoids

- Heterotropic bone
- Ingrown toenail
- Insect bites
- Intestinal distention
- Invasive testing
- Menstruation
- Pain
- Pregnancy: labor and delivery
- Pressure ulcers
- Pulmonary emboli
- Scrotal compression
- Sexual intercourse
- Surgical incision (skin)
- Surgical or diagnostic procedures
- Temperature fluctuations
- Urinary tract infection
- Urodynamics
- Uterine contractions
- Vaginitis

Medical Management

Onset of autonomic hyperreflexia is a medical emergency. Medical management begins with thoroughly educating the patient, family, and/or caregivers to recognize the signs and symptoms of autonomic hyperreflexia and to initiate appropriate treatment measures as quickly and efficiently as possible to prevent dangerous sequelae. The initial treatment measure is removal of the causative stimulus, if at all possible. Symptoms that persist despite stimulus removal require pharmacologic intervention, the main form of which is reduction of the hypertension that has been precipitated.

Complications

If left untreated, the sustained peripheral hypertension can culminate in serious sequelae, such as retinal hemorrhage, myocardial infarction, cerebral hemorrhage, seizures, hypertensive crisis, stroke, and death.

Anesthesia Implications

Because this unregulated sympathetic response to stimulation occurs rapidly, the primary concern of the anesthetist is to provide adequate depth of anesthesia. Essentially any method of anesthesia is acceptable—general, regional, or local infiltration—provided the depth of anesthesia ameliorates the reflexive response to surgical stimulation. General anesthesia is the easiest method of achieving a depth adequate to prevent reflexive response to stimulation. Epidural or subarachnoid anesthesia is an appropriate anesthetic choice. However, it can be difficult for the following reasons: (1) determination of the level of anesthesia is inexact, at best; and (2) technical difficulties arise because of vertebral deformities, osteoporosis, and positioning. Regional anesthesia is capable of blocking the afferent pathways to prevent the sympathetic discharge, but once "set," the level or depth cannot be changed. General anesthesia is the only technique whereby the depth can be deepened to thwart the onset of unopposed sympathetic response to surgical stimulation; epidural anesthesia levels (if obtained at all) can be adjusted, but in a much more limited manner.

Barrett's Esophagus

B

Definition

Barrett's esophagus (BE) is a peptic ulcer in the lower esophagus, often associated with stricture, caused by the presence of columnar-lined epithelium. The columnar-lined epithelium may contain functional mucous cells, parietal cells, or chief cells in the esophagus instead of the normal squamous cell epithelium. The presence of specialized intestinal metaplasia (SIM) with goblet cells confirms the diagnosis of BE.

Incidence

The incidence is divided into two subtypes: long-segment Barrett's esophagus (LSBE) and short-segment Barrett's esophagus (SSBE). In LSBE, the incidence is reported to be 0.3% to 2% of the entire population, but 8% to 20% in patients with gastroesophageal reflex disease (GERD). In the United States, the incidence is 376:100,000, predominately in Caucasian males. In SSBE, the incidence is reported to be 5% to 30%.

Etiology

BE is a complication of GERD. Patients who develop BE usually have a combination of symptoms. Prolonged esophageal acid fixation produces erosive esophagitis. The pH of the refluxate, combined with the duration of contact with the esophageal mucosa, determines the degree of mucosal injury. Prolonged exposure erodes the esophageal mucosa, promotes inflammatory cellular infiltrates, and can culminate in epithelial necrosis. The damage and necrosis lead to replacement of the damaged tissue with metaplastic columnar cells, the origin of which is not understood. Patients with LSBE generally have longer durations of reflux symptoms, severe combined patterns of reflux (in both supine and erect positions), and low pressure at the lower esophageal sphincter (LES). LSBE patients are less sensitive to direct acid exposure to the esophagus. SSBE patients have a greater sensitivity to direct acid exposure to the esophagus, shorter duration of reflux, and only upright (erect) reflux.

B

Signs and Symptoms

- Acid regurgitation
- Delayed esophageal acid clearance time
- Duodenogastric reflux
- Dysphagia (occasional)

- Hiatal hernia
- Pyrosis
- Reduced lower esophageal sphincter tone

Medical Management

BE does not warrant a specific therapeutic regimen. Treatment is primarily for the associated GERD, which entails use of histamine (H_2)-receptor antagonists and proton pump inhibitors (PPIs). PPIs may prove more advantageous than the H_2-receptor antagonists because of the relative insensitivity of patients with BE to esophageal acid. Dietary alterations are also part of the treatment regimen, such as elimination of fatty foods, fried foods, chocolate, alcohol, coffee, and citrus fruit or juices. Weight loss and smoking cessation are also of great importance in the treatment of BE. Surgical treatments, such as Nissen fundoplication, do not reverse BE nor do they halt or prevent the progression to development of esophageal cancer. Periodic endoscopic evaluations are needed to monitor the progression of the disease.

Complications

If left unchecked, BE can progress to esophageal cancer. This occurs in approximately 0.5% of cases. When dysplasia is high grade, the standard treatment is surgical esophagectomy. Other complications include esophageal perforation, mediastinitis, and hemorrhage.

Anesthesia Implications

The GERD associated with BE is the primary concern for anesthetists. A rapid sequence induction should be performed. Before anesthesia, the patient should be advised to continue the routine for taking the PPI, especially along with the H_2-receptor he or she has been prescribed.

The use of local anesthetic agents, such as bupivacaine, mepivacaine, and lidocaine should be undertaken with caution because of the increased risk of anesthetic toxicity.

Bartter Syndrome

Definition

Bartter syndrome is a form of hyperaldosteronism that results from hypertrophy and hyperplasia of the juxtaglomerular cells, with normal blood pressure and hyperkalemic alkalosis without edema, increased renin concentration, angiotension II, and bradykinin. It is the manifestation of one of three genetic expressions: neonatal Bartter syndrome, classic Bartter syndrome, and Gitelman syndrome.

Incidence

Bartter syndrome is extremely rare. The precise incidence is not known. The disease process is seen worldwide, with no exclusion of race and approximately equal occurrence in both sexes. The neonatal form is typically known before birth, whereas diagnosis of the classic form is typically made within the first 2 years of life.

Etiology

Bartter syndrome predominately occurs as neonatal or classic forms. Neonatal Bartter syndrome (NBS) is subdivided into two types: type I NBS comes from a mutation in the sodium chloride/potassium chloride co-transporter gene; type II NBS comes from mutations in the ROMK gene. Classic Bartter syndrome develops as a result of mutation(s) in the chloride-channel gene (CIC-kb).

In each of these three subtypes a large volume of urine that is high in sodium, potassium, and chloride is delivered to the distal segments of the renal tubules. In that area only sodium is reabsorbed while potassium is secreted.

The characteristics of the disease are hypokalemia, hypochloremia, metabolic acidosis, and hyperreninemia (while the blood pressure remains normal). In both types of Bartter syndrome, classic and neonatal, the sentinel histologic finding is hyperplasia of the juxtaglomerular apparatus. Other histologic findings are listed in the box on the following page.

B

Histologic Findings in the Patient with Bartter Syndrome

- Apical vacuolization of proximal tubular cells
- Glomerular hyalinization
- Interstitial fibrosis
- Juxtaglomerular apparatus hyperplasia
- Medullary interstitial cells hyperplasia (infrequent finding)
- Tubular atrophy

Signs and Symptoms

Neonatal Bartter Syndrome
- Maternal polyhydramnios
- Neonate with massive polyuria (12 to 50 mL/kg/hr)
- Preterm delivery
- Secondary fetal polyuria

Classic Bartter Syndrome
- Constipation
- Cramps
- Developmental delays
- Failure to thrive
- Fatigue
- History of maternal polyhydramnios
- Linear growth retardation
- Minimal brain dysfunction
- Muscle weakness
- Nonspecific electroencephalographic changes
- Polydipsia
- Polyuria
- Preterm delivery
- Recurrent carpopedal spasms
- Salt craving
- Volume depletion
- Vomiting

Medical Management

Correction of dehydration is important, along with "realignment" of electrolyte values. The patient with NBS is frequently treated with indomethacin combined with potassium supplementation. The patient with classic Bartter syndrome is treated with potassium supplements, which are frequently insufficient; potassium-sparing diuretics may be added with only transient effects. The best method for correction of hypokalemia is administration of prostaglandin synthetase inhibitors. The patient, no matter what age, is encouraged to take in food and drink rich in potassium, such as bananas, citrus fruits and juices, tomatoes, and skim milk. The patient's activity level is typically not restricted; however, the possibility of dehydration must be closely monitored. Strenuous exercise should be avoided because of the increased probability of dehydration, exacerbation of potassium loss created by the dehydration, and the increased potential for functional cardiac dysfunction/dysrhythmias secondary to the excessive potassium loss.

Complications

Failure to thrive, growth retardation, and developmental delays occur in pediatric patients (neonatal or classic Bartter syndrome) if symptomatic treatment is not instituted. Dehydration can exacerbate electrolyte imbalances and produce cardiac dysrhythmias and/or sudden cardiac death. Chronic hypokalemia progresses over time to culminate in chronic renal insufficiency and/or renal failure.

Anesthesia Implications

For the anesthetist the primary focus for a patient with Bartter syndrome should be on the fluid status and electrolyte levels, particularly in procedures with expected large volumes of blood loss, insensitive fluid losses, and third-spacing of fluids. The patient with Bartter syndrome is particularly prone to dehydration and hypokalemia. A good recommendation would be to place a second, large-bore intravenous line to facilitate rapid fluid administration if necessary. Also, a secondary infusion containing supplemental potassium chloride (KCl) may be appropriate.

Chronic hypokalemia may contribute to delayed gastric emptying, so it should be assumed that the patient has a full stomach at the time of induction. The patient with Bartter syndrome is more prone to develop an ileus, therefore gastric evacuation may be appropriate after the airway is secured. To help minimize the potassium losses from this source, it may be more appropriate to allow gastric fluids to drain via gravity rather than external suction. The best course of action might be to leave the nasogastric tube in place without suction or gravity drainage until a need is indicated by a feeling of nausea and/or very slow to absent bowel sounds.

B

Chronic hypokalemia can have an impact on the patient's response to and recovery from neuromuscular blocking agents. It may also contribute to the presence of cardiac dysrhythmias and alter the activity of baroreceptors.

Hyperventilation may exacerbate both the hypokalemia and metabolic acidosis already present.

Because the patient with Bartter syndrome often has a history of treatment with prostaglandin inhibitors, the patient may be resistant to the effects of vasopressors.

Becker's Dystrophy

Definition

Becker's dystrophy is a genetic variation of Duchenne's muscular dystrophy. This form is very similar to pseudohypertrophic muscular dystrophy (Duchenne's), but the onset of the disease occurs later in life and progresses more slowly. However, the ultimate debilitation is the same as with Duchenne's.

Incidence

The Becker's dystrophy phenotype occurs at a rate of approximately 24:1,000,000 population. The onset may occur any time from 3 years of age through adulthood, even late adulthood.

Etiology

The genotype for Becker's dystrophy is the result of a sex-linked transmission on the X chromosome in the Xp 21 stripe. The Becker phenotype correlates with point mutations that preserve reading frame or genetic deletions that cause less structural compromise.

Signs and Symptoms

- Age, usually 10 to 20 years
- Calf enlargement
- Gait disturbances
- Kyphoscoliosis
- Progressive development of muscle weakness
- Progressive diminishment of deep tendon reflexes
- Waning forced vital capacity and other lung volumes

Medical Management

Prednisone is currently the only medication that has demonstrated any benefit in the treatment of Becker's dystrophy. The dose is 0.75 to 1.5 mg/kg/day in divided doses. The muscle wasting produced by this disease is retarded or delayed by the administration of prednisone. The benefit of prednisone administration may become evident as soon as 1 month after initiation of treatment, but those benefits generally last only about 3 years. These benefits may also be somewhat diminished by sequelae resulting from chronic steroid administration.

The remainder of medical management of Becker's dystrophy concentrates on measures and strategies to maximize functional status, maintain muscle tone, and delay reliance on a wheelchair for as long as possible. Exercising joints and stretching muscles daily can delay the onset of debilitating contractures. These exercises work synergistically with the application of various supportive braces, such as ankle-foot or knee-ankle-foot orthoses, to help maintain the ability to stand, whether mobile or not, and further contribute to the delay of debilitating contractures and scoliosis.

Becker's dystrophy is a progressive disease that ultimately culminates in muscle-joint contractures, profound muscle weakness, and disability. When the patient becomes wheelchair dependent, the possibility of developing pressure sores increases. This possibility is further exacerbated by the chronic administration of corticosteroids. With the development of pressure sores comes the greater potential for infection and sepsis. Muscle wasting or atrophy and weakness contribute to alteration in pulmonary function, particularly forced vital capacity (FVC). Diminished pulmonary function can lead to the development of atelectasis and pneumonia. Frequent use of incentive spirometry can help prevent atelectasis and pneumonia. The decline in pulmonary function may necessitate some manner of ventilatory support, ranging from noninvasive, such as continuous positive airway pressure (CPAP), to minimally invasive, such as bilevel positive airway pressure (BiPAP), to invasive, such as tracheal intubation or tracheostomy, with or without mechanical ventilation. Tracheal intubation should be a short-term measure that should be supplanted by tracheostomy, whether or not it is combined with mechanical ventilation.

The sequelae of chronic steroid administration can contribute to the development of complications. The patient who depends on steroids may be more susceptible to skin breakdown and infection, whether via pressure sore or the pulmonary system, as well as weight gain and cushingoid habitus. The weight gain and cushingoid habitus may further exacerbate the potential for pressure sore development, infection, and diminution of pulmonary function.

Dystrophin is found not only in the skeletal muscle, but also in significant quantity in the cardiac and brain tissues. Pseudo-hypertrophy may also occur in the heart muscle tissue, leading to cardiac fibrosis, which results in reduced cardiac output with ensuing pulmonary congestion, spiraling downward to fulminate congestive heart failure. Cardiac fibrosis also affects the cardiac conduction system. Fibrotic changes in cardiac conduction may be evidenced by tall R waves in the V_1 lead, deep Q waves in the AVL, AVR, and AVF leads, shortened P-R interval, and sinus tachycardia. As a result, lethal dysrhythmias may occur. Loss of dystrophin from cerebral tissue leads to developmental delays and diminished intellectual development. There is a shift to the left with regard to intelligence quotient (IQ) distribution; the mean IQ has been reported at 83.

Complications

- Atelectasis
- Cardiac conduction abnormalities
- Cardiac fibrosis
- Congestive heart failure
- Cushingoid habitus
- Decline in pulmonary function
- Developmental delays, diminished intellectual development
- Infection
- Muscle wasting or atrophy
- Pneumonia
- Pressure sores
- Pseudohypertrophy (skeletal and/or cardiac muscle)
- Sepsis
- Weight gain

Anesthesia Implications

Preoperative pulmonary function testing is appropriate to assess the degree of incapacity the disease has produced, and it contributes to the decision as to which anesthetic technique to use and whether the patient will require ventilatory support postoperatively. For the patient with severely diminished pulmonary function, regional anesthesia—specifically subarachnoid or epidural—may not be appropriate. A severe decline in pulmonary function implies severe muscle weakness, especially of the accessory muscles of breathing (intercostal and sterno-cleidomastoid muscles), which may be further exacerbated by instillation of such a regional technique. The work of breathing may quickly overwhelm the patient's already limited energy reserves. Periods of postoperative respiratory embarrassment or dysfunction may be drawn out by as much as 36 hours, even though the patient's muscle strength may appear to recover to the same level as observed preoperatively.

Heart failure is a real possibility during anesthesia, particularly for major surgical procedures, despite normal results on preoperative electrocardiogram and echocardiogram. Stress echocardiography using angiotensin has been advocated to detect latent heart failure and to identify any contraction abnormalities that may be induced.

Administration of anesthesia medications requires much consideration. Malignant hyperthermia (MH)–like symptoms may occur in the patient with Becker's dystrophy, as well as in those with other muscular dystrophies. The potent inhalational agents are not recommended—nor is succinylcholine—in the patient with Becker's dystrophy because of the potential production of MH-like symptoms, including rhabdomyolysis. Inhalation agents may also exacerbate any cardiac dysfunction that may be present or induce latent dysfunction. Hypnotics must also be selected judiciously. Thiopental may be used, but the doses must be significantly reduced. Propofol may be preferable to all others, but the induction dose may be larger than anticipated; moreover, administration of propofol must be closely scrutinized relative to the patient's functional myocardial status because of the high degree of myocardial depression propofol produces. Parenteral narcotic analgesics may be used to supplant the need for potent inhalational agents. However, the choice of opiate must take into account the need for postoperative ventilation. Therefore shorter-acting opiates, such as alfentanil or remifentanil, may be more appropriate. Nondepolarizing muscle relaxants are likely to demonstrate increases in both effect as well as duration of action. Recovery from nondepolarizing muscle relaxants has been reported to be as much as three to six times longer than usually expected. The patient with Becker's dystrophy—as well as those with all muscular dystrophies—experience abnormalities of smooth muscle. The combination of these abnormalities, inactivity, and general anesthesia may delay gastric emptying, thus increasing the potential for regurgitation and aspiration during induction/intubation and emergence/extubation.

Behçet's Disease

Definition

Behçet's disease is believed to be an autoimmune disorder characterized by uveitis and retinal vasculitis, optic atrophy, and aphthous lesions of the mouth and genitalia. Frequently there are other signs and symptoms that suggest diffuse vasculitis. Actual signs and symptoms vary according to the organ system involved.

Incidence

The incidence of Behçet's disease varies according to ethnicity. The highest incidences are among Middle Eastern and Far Eastern populations.

Incidence of Behçet's Disease (per 100,000)	
United States	0.3-6.6
Turkey	370
United Kingdom	0.64
Saudi Arabia	20
Iran	16-100
Japan	13.5
Germany	2

Etiology

Behçet's disease is believed t o be of autoimmune origin. As such, the true etiology remains unknown. Various aspects of the disease seem to indicate that it is an infectious process, but in the 80 years since it was first described, no specific causative agent has been identified. Genetic factors also seem to contribute to the development of this disease. Middle and Far Eastern populations have a higher rate of occurrence of this disease and have a higher prevalence of human leukocyte antigen B_5 (HLA-B_5); the Israeli population has a higher prevalence of HLA-$B_5$1.

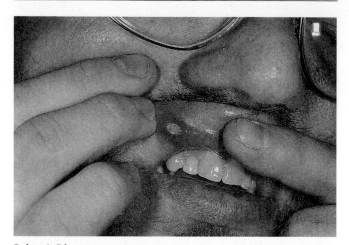

Behçet's Disease. Oral aphthous lesions in a patient with Behçet's disease.
(From Callen JP, et al: Dermatological Signs of Internal Disease, *ed. 3, Philadelphia, 2003, Saunders.)*

Signs and Symptoms

Arthritis
- Enthesopathies
- Joint fluid turbidity
- Sacroilitis

Cardiac
- Coronary thrombosis
- Coronary vasculitis
- Diastolic dysfunction
- Endocarditis
- Myocarditis
- Pericarditis
- Valvular regurgitation

Gastrointestinal
- Abdominal pain
- Bloody diarrhea
- Intestinal perforation
- Ulcerative lesions

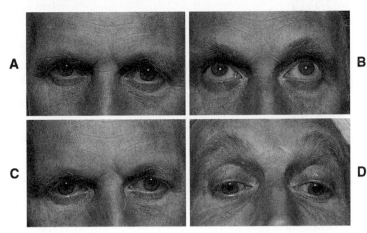

Behçet's Disease. Failure of horizontal gaze (**A** and **C**) associated with preservation of vertical gaze (**B** and **D**). *(From Perkin GD:* Mosby's Color Atlas and Text of Neurology, *ed. 2, Edinburgh, 2002, Mosby.)*

Genitalia
- Penile lesions
- Perianal lesions
- Scrotal lesions
- Vulvar/vaginal lesions

Mouth
- Aphthous lesions/ulcers

Neurologic (10% to 30% of cases)
- Acute deafness
- Behavioral changes
- Clonus
- Cranial nerve lesions
- Dementia
- Emotional liability
- Meningoencephalitis
- Positive Babinski sign
- Seizures
- Spastic paralysis/pyramidal tract lesions
- Speech difficulty
- Swallowing difficulty

B

Ocular
- Anterior uveitis
- Cataracts
- Glaucoma
- Hypopyon
- Infarctions
- Posterior uveitis
- Retinal detachment
- Retinal edema
- Retinal vasculitis
- Synechiae

Pulmonary
- Hemoptysis
- Pleural effusions
- Pulmonary hypertension
- Pulmonary vasculitis

Renal
- Epididymitis
- Glomerulonephritis
- Immunoglobin A nephropathy

Skin
- Erythema nodosum
- Pseudofolliculitis
- Pustular, acnelike lesions

Vascular
- Aneurysms
- Claudication
- Ischemia
- Myocardial infarction
- Thrombotic disease
- Transient ischemic attack
- Vasculitis

Medical Management

Management of Behçet's disease varies according to the organ system(s) involved:

Central nervous system: Typically treated with prednisone or prednisolone, chlorambucil, or cyclophosphamide.

Erythema nodosum: Treatment is generally with colchicine or dapsone.

Gastrointestinal system: Treating lesions in this system is usually accomplished using corticosteroids, sulfasalazine, or thalidomide.

Joints: Localized intra-articular injections of corticosteroids, prednisone, and/or nonsteroidal anti-inflammatory drugs (NSAIDs) may be used for treatment of joint pain.

Colchicine, sulfasalazine, interferon-Q, levamisole, and
azathioprine may also be utilized.

Ophthalmic manifestations: Topical drops, consisting of both
mydriatic and corticosteroid medications, are utilized.
Immunosuppression is attempted because of the autoimmune nature of the disease and is generally achieved using azathioprine, systemic corticosteroids, cyclosporine,
chlorambucil, tacrolimus, or cyclophosphamide.

Systemic manifestations (skin disease or severe ulcers): Colchicine or azathioprine is used with some degree of success. Antileprosy drugs, such as dapsone and thalidomide
along with the immune system–modifying drug levamisole, have demonstrated varying degrees of usefulness.

Thrombosis/thrombotic events: Anticoagulants are the treatment of choice.

Vasculitis: Immunosuppression is the treatment goal, utilizing suppressive medications such as cyclophosphamide,
azathioprine, cyclosporine, and others. If anticoagulants
are required in the treatment of pulmonary vasculitis, the
mortality of patients may be increased.

Tumor necrosis factor antagonists, such as etanercept or infliximab, have demonstrated efficacy in treating Behçet's disease.

Surgical intervention may be required to treat a variety of
manifestations of Behçet's disease, including gastrointestinal
perforation(s) and the resulting peritonitis, aneurysms, endo-
cardial fibrosis, coronary thrombosis, glaucoma, cataracts, and
retinal detachment.

Complications

Three manifestations of Behçet's disease can be especially
devastating: aneurysms, thrombolic events, and vasculitis.
Aneurysms may develop essentially at any location: thoracic,
abdominal, cranial, ophthalmic, or the extremities. The effects,
should an aneurysm rupture, can range from vision impairment
and/or loss to death.

Anesthesia Implications

As with any patient, a thorough preoperative history is
indispensable. Prior knowledge that the patient has Behçet's
disease should prompt heightened concentration on and

investigation of all organ systems. Magnetic resonance imaging (MRI) or computed tomography (CT) may be warranted to assess for possible spinal cord compression, intracranial pressure increases, or intervertebral disk herniation. Initial cardiac manifestations may be indicated by electrocardiography and echocardiography. Potential pulmonary manifestations may necessitate arterial blood gas analysis, chest x-ray, spirometry, and pulmonary function testing. Renal involvement may be initially assessed via laboratory determination of blood urea nitrogen (BUN) and creatinine concentrations, particularly for the patient being treated with NSAIDs and/or antineoplastic medications. Prophylactic steroid coverage is necessary for the patient being treated with corticosteroids.

The patient with an autoimmune disorder may experience an exacerbation as a result of any skin puncture, such as insertion of an intravenous line or arterial pressure line or instillation of a regional anesthetic. Securing the patient's airway during administration of general anesthesia can be a considerable challenge.

Direct laryngoscopy or placement of a laryngeal mask airway (LMA) can aggravate and rupture lesions that may be present in the mouth and/or oropharynx, producing significant bleeding. The patient treated with NSAIDs and/or anticoagulants may experience even greater blood loss. The risk versus benefit of continuing these classes of medications within 7 to 10 hours of a surgical procedure must be given consideration. Lesions in the oropharynx may extend to and into the glottis and trachea, resulting in glottic stenosis, which will make passage of an endotracheal tube more difficult. If the stenosis is severe enough, intubation may only be achieved by fiberoptic means; however, if intubation proves impossible, a surgical tracheostomy may be necessary to secure the airway to provide anesthesia for the surgical intervention(s) that are required. The patient may be more susceptible to pulmonary injury in the form of barotrauma, particularly if the patient has pulmonary vasculitis. The patient may benefit considerably from pressure-controlled ventilation rather than volume-controlled ventilation.

Beta Thalassemia

Definition

Beta thalassemia is an inherited blood disease of abnormal hemoglobin production in which both beta-globin subunit components of normal hemoglobin are absent.

Incidence

The estimated incidence rates of beta thalassemia vary by population and it is more commonly found in areas around the Mediterranean Sea; in Italian, Sicilian, and Greek populations, the incidence is approximately 10%; in African populations, it is approximately 1.5%; in the African American population, the incidence is approximately 1.5%; and in Southeastern Asian populations, it is approximately 5%.

Etiology

The manufacture of beta-globin molecules has been traced to chromosome 11. More than 200 mutations of the beta-globin genes on chromosome 11 that can result in thalassemia have been documented. The result of the particular mutation is either the absence of the beta-globin, called beta(0)thalassemia, or diminished beta-globin, called beta(+) thalassemia.

Signs and Symptoms

- Abdominal swelling
- Amenorrhea
- Cardiac failure
- Cardiomegaly
- Dark urine
- Dysrhythmias
- Facial deformities
- Failure to grow/thrive
- Frontal bossing
- Gallstones
- Infection
- Irritability
- Jaundice
- Leg ulcers
- Mongoloid facies
- Pallor
- Progressive hepatospleno-megaly
- Severe anemia
- Sexual development retardation
- Skeletal deformities

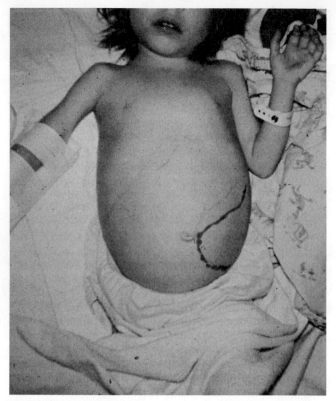

Beta Thalassemia. A child with beta thalassemia major who has severe splenomegaly. *(From Jorde LB, et al:* Medical Genetics *[updated for 2006-2007], ed. 3, St Louis, 2006, Mosby.)*

Medical Management

The primary goal of treatment is to achieve and maintain correction of the anemia. Anemia is evident by 6 months of age as the neonate's physiology converts from fetal hemoglobin to adult hemoglobin. The patient becomes dependent on transfusions very early in life and remains transfusion-dependent for his or her entire life. The patient should be placed on a regular schedule of transfusion. The transfusion protocols are classified as conservative, hypertransfusion, and supertransfusion (see box on p. 57). The hypertransfusion

Transfusion Protocols for the Patient with Beta Thalassemia

- *Conservative:* Transfuse when the hemoglobin level is >6 to 8 g/dL or the patient becomes symptomatic.
- *Hypertransfusion:* Transfuse frequently enough to ensure the hemoglobin level is maintained at >10 g/dL and the hematocrit is >30%. Proper hemoglobin level maintenance also suppresses endogenous erythroid activity, prevents bone marrow expansion, and reduces absorption of dietary iron. This method is associated with a high incidence of hemosiderosis.
- *Supertransfusion:* Transfuse frequently enough to achieve and maintain a hematocrit level >35%; usually two or three units are transfused every 2 to 4 weeks. This method is also associated with a high incidence of hemosiderosis.

regimen has the secondary benefit of reducing the patient's ineffective erythropoiesis.

The patient with beta thalassemia should receive broad-spectrum antibiotics after febrile illnesses, based on the results of urine and/or blood cultures. The patient who has undergone splenectomy frequently receives prophylactic penicillin therapy.

The only treatment option currently available that is considered to be potentially curative is bone marrow transplantation. Other therapies being investigated and evaluated include augmentation of fetal hemoglobin synthesis, bisphosphonate therapies, and gene therapy.

Surgical interventions related to beta thalassemia are limited. Typical surgical interventions are placement of permanent, indwelling central venous catheter(s) and splenectomy. Splenectomy is frequently avoidable if the child is maintained on an aggressive transfusion protocol and should be delayed or deferred until the patient is older than 6 years of age to minimize the potential of overwhelming infection.

Complications

- Aplastic and megaloblastic crises
- Cholelithiasis
- Chronic hemolysis
- Death
- Delayed/absent puberty
- Heart failure
- Hemolytic anemia
- Hepatic siderosis
- Impaired growth rate

- Iron overload
- Pathologic fractures
- Septicemia

- Severe anemia
- Splenomegaly

Anesthesia Implications

The patient with beta thalassemia may present to the operating room with significant anemia, depending on where he or she is in the transfusion protocol. The degree of anemia dictates this patient's O_2-carrying capacity. The anesthetist should strive to optimize the patient's O_2-carrying capabilities by performing preoperative and/or perioperative transfusion(s) and providing as close to 100% oxygen as possible for the anesthetic. Preoperative complete blood count and basic metabolic panel are imperative laboratory studies for the patient with beta thalassemia.

The anesthetist must be very discerning with regard to the liver function test results. The patient with beta thalassemia is prone to develop hemochromatosis secondary to the multiple transfusions received throughout his or her lifetime. As a result of the induced liver dysfunction, metabolism may be prolonged for a host of anesthesia-related drugs, from opiates to hypnotics to benzodiazepines to muscle relaxants. The anesthetist may need to reduce the doses of these drugs. If the liver dysfunction becomes severe enough, the patient may experience coagulation irregularities. The anesthetist may need to administer coagulation adjuncts, such as vitamin K or various coagulation factors or fresh frozen plasma. As a result, the anesthetist should anticipate greater than expected blood volume losses for a given surgical intervention.

Beta thalassemia causes bone marrow hyperplasia and accelerated hematopoiesis. The hematopoiesis acceleration produces distortion of some of the bones, most notably distortion of the craniofacial bones. The patient with beta thalassemia is characterized by the "chipmunk" face that results from the craniofacial anatomy distortion. Cranial radiographs demonstrate what is known as "hair-on-end" patterns. The craniofacial distortions produced by beta thalassemia may make direct laryngoscopy more difficult than would otherwise be anticipated.

The patient with beta thalassemia is prone to pathologic fractures. As a result, the anesthetist must take great care during the process of positioning the patient and ensure adequate padding to bony prominences. Because of their greater ability to disperse pressure, gelatin-filled pads are superior to foam padding.

> **Budd-Chiari Syndrome**

Definition

Budd-Chiari syndrome is an uncommon condition of obstruction of intrahepatic veins. It is induced by thrombotic or non-thrombotic obstruction of hepatic venous outflow, leading to congestive hepatopathy. The hepatopathy results from large and small vein obstruction of venous outflow, producing hepatocellular injury from microvascular ischemia. It eventually results in portal hypertension and then liver insufficiency and failure.

Incidence

Exact incidence of Budd-Chiari syndrome is not known; it is classified as a rare entity both in the United States and internationally.

Etiology

Budd-Chiari syndrome frequently occurs in patients who already have some manner of thrombotic diathesis, including myeloproliferative disorders, pregnancy, tumors, chronic inflammatory diseases, clotting disorders, and infections.

Causes of Budd-Chiari Syndrome	
Chronic Infections • Amoebic abscess • Aspergillosis • Hydatid cysts • Syphilis • Tuberculosis **Chronic Inflammatory Diseases** • Behçet's disease (see p. 49) • Inflammatory bowel disease • Sarcoidosis • Sjögren syndrome (see p. 316) • Systemic lupus erythematosus (see p. 335)	**Hematologic Disorders** • Antiphospholipid antibody syndrome • Essential thrombocytosis • Paroxysmal nocturnal hemoglobinuria • Polycythemia rubra vera • Unspecified myeloproliferative disorder

Continued

Causes of Budd-Chiari Syndrome—cont'd

Inherited Thrombotic Diathesis
- Antithrombin III deficiency
- Factor V Leiden deficiency
- Membranous web
- Oral contraceptives
- Pregnancy/postpartum
- Protein C deficiency
- Protein S deficiency

Tumors
- Hepatocellular carcinoma
- Leiomyosarcoma
- Renal cell carcinoma
- Right atrial myoma
- Wilms' tumor

Miscellaneous
- α_1-Antitrypsin deficiency
- Dacarbazine
- Idiopathic causes
- Trauma
- Urethane exposure

Signs and Symptoms

- Abdominal distention
- Acute right upper quadrant pain
- Age of onset: 40 to 50 years
- Ascites
- Engorgement of vessels of chest and abdominal walls
- Polycythemia vera
- Prolonged prothrombin time
- Splenomegaly
- Tender hepatomegaly

Medical Management

Most patients present with a classic symptom triad: abdominal pain, ascites, and hepatomegaly. However, this triad is nonspecific and making the diagnosis of this disease requires that one have a high index of suspicion when the patient exhibits this symptom triad. There are four clinical variants: acute liver disease, subacute liver disease, fulminate liver disease, and liver failure. The most common variant is subacute liver failure with portal hypertension and liver decompensation.

Medical therapy can be instituted for short-term, symptomatic relief. The mortality rate associated with symptomatic treatment is 80% to 85%. Treatment includes anticoagulation, antithrombolytic therapy, and angioplasty. Ascites can be managed with sodium restriction and diuretics, with approximately 95% effectiveness. In the event of hypotension, water restriction may be incorporated. Paracentesis may be used for some patients, but it is typically reserved for the patient with tense ascites in whom rapid symptomatic relief is needed. Invasive/surgical intervention can be undertaken for decompression of the hepatic vascular congestion if portal hypertension is the underlying cause of symptoms. Peritoneovenous shunt placement is an older, almost obsolete, therapeutic measure for symptomatic relief of medically intractable ascites. The placement of this shunt can result in increased cardiac output, renal blood flow, glomerular filtration rate, urinary volume, sodium excretion, and decreased plasma renin activity and plasma aldosterone concentration. There is no evidence of improved patient survival. Currently, the emerging standard treatment is the transjugular intrahepatic portosystemic shunt (TIPS) for alleviation of the hepatic venous congestion. Prognosis for this disease can be good, based on several factors.

Complications

- Electrolyte imbalance
- Hepatic decompensation
- Hepatic encephalopathy
- Hepatorenal syndrome
- Hypercoagulation state
- Intravascular volume shifts (for large volume paracentesis)
- Portal hypertension
- Spontaneous bacterial peritonitis
- Variceal hemorrhage

Anesthesia Implications

The liver receives 25% to 30% of the cardiac output when at rest. Approximately 75% of the hepatic blood flow is delivered via the portal vein. The portal system delivers 35% to 50% of the oxygen the liver receives; the remaining 50% to 65% is delivered by the hepatic artery. Portal hypertension associated with Budd-Chiari syndrome is post-sinusoidal intrahepatic in nature. The circumvention of the metabolic processing provided by the hepatocytes may produce a prolongation and exaggeration of the effects of a large number

B

of anesthesia-related drugs, particularly those with high hepatic extraction rates.

Preoperative electrolyte balance and coagulation parameters should be ascertained. Ascites formation and its removal can result in larger shifts in the electrolytes levels. The patient with Budd-Chiari syndrome may be treated with anticoagulants and/or antithrombolytic agents. As a result, the level of treatment must be assessed and adjustments made before any elective procedure. Obviously, liver function testing is an essential preoperative evaluation. Reduced albumin levels can result in increased bioavailability of a large number of drugs.

Cardiopulmonary function should be thoroughly assessed preoperatively. Over time, liver function with ascites formation can produce transudative effusions, usually on the right side initially. Communication between the pleural and peritoneal spaces can allow ascites fluid to accumulate in the pleural cavity, causing decreased pulmonary compliance, reduced lung volumes, and elevated pleural pressures. As a result, moderate hypoxemia may ensue.

Choanal Atresia

Definition

Choanal atresia is the congenital absence or closure of the paired openings between the nasal cavity and the nasopharynx. Because this obstruction is complete, the neonate with choanal atresia becomes an obligatory nose breather. The condition can cause death by asphyxiation in the newborn.

Incidence

The average incidence of choanal atresia is 0.82:10,000. Unilateral involvement occurs more frequently than the bilateral form by a ratio of about 2:1, with the right side being affected more often than the left. This condition affects females more frequently than males.

Etiology

During the normal uterine developmental process, the nasal cavities extend posteriorly under the influence of the posteriorly directed fusion of the palatal processes. The membrane thins, separating the nasal cavities from the oral cavity. The two-layer membrane that consists of nasal and oral epithelia ruptures and forms the choanae. This occurs by the 38th developmental day. If this rupture fails to occur, choanal atresia is the result. The "preliminary" choanae are not in the same location as the definitive choanae, which are eventually located even more posteriorly.

Signs and Symptoms

- Alleviation of respiratory distress by crying
- Arched hard palate
- Bilateral rhinorrhea
- Components of CHARGE (see box)
- Cyclical cyanosis
- Medialized lateral nasal well
- Narrow nasopharynx
- Severe airway obstruction
- Unilateral rhinorrhea
- Widened vomer

Medical Management

Choanal atresia is treated chiefly by surgical correction of the congenital anomaly. Bony involvement is present in 90% of patients. Bilateral atresia is generally corrected in the neonatal period. The surgical procedure is performed via a transnasal approach using either the CO_2 or Nd:YAG (neodymium: yttrium-aluminum-garnet) laser. Stents are placed in the newly created nasal passages for 3 to 5 weeks to maintain patency and improve continued postoperative passage patency. For the patient with unilateral atresia, definitive diagnosis may not occur for several years. Surgical correction should not be undertaken at any time during childhood.

Complications

- Aspiration
- Neonatal demise (from bilateral atresia)
- Respiratory arrest

Anesthesia Implications

Age-appropriate implications and concerns are foremost for infants and very young children scheduled for any surgical procedure. Corrective surgery for choanal atresia is no different.

Airway management may be difficult. Infants with CHARGE association should have their cardiac function thoroughly evaluated preoperatively.

CHARGE Association
Coloboma of the iris, choroid, and/or microphthalmia
Heart defect
Atresia of the choanae
Retarded growth and development
Genitourinary abnormalities (cryptorchidism, microphallus, hydronephrosis)
Ear defects associated with deafness

Co-morbidities or other associated abnormalities must be carefully considered and evaluated preoperatively.

The airway should be secured using an oral RAE tube after either inhalational or intravenous induction, whichever is more age appropriate.

Craniosynostosis Malformations

- Antley-Bixler syndrome*
- Apert syndrome (acrocephalosyndactyly)*
- Crouzon syndrome (craniofacial dysostosis)*
- Pfeiffer syndrome (Pfeiffer-type acrocephalosyndactyly)*
- Saethre-Chotzen syndrome*

*See Appendix G: Rare Syndromes.

The patient should be extubated while as awake as possible with intact protective reflexes robust. However, if the surgical procedure has been prolonged, there may be significant airway edema and/or hemodynamic instability. In that case, the patient should remain intubated and sedated to allow for resolution of any such concerns before extubating and increasing the potential for catastrophic airway compromise.

Churg-Strauss Syndrome

Definition

Churg-Strauss syndrome (CSS) is an allergic, granulomatous angitis that is a variant of necrotizing vasculitis in which there is significant lung involvement. It also affects the musculoskeletal, cardiac, and peripheral nervous systems. CSS is sometimes referred to as polyarteritis nodosa with lung involvement.

Incidence

The true incidence of CSS is uncertain, but it is less frequent than classic polyarteritis nodosa. It has been documented in all age groups but is extremely rare among infants.

Etiology

The etiology of CSS is unknown; however, there is a strong association with allergic diathesis and frequently severe and/or intractable asthma.

Signs and Symptoms

- Cerebral infarcts
- Congestive heart failure
- Coronary vasculitis
- Cutaneous nodules
- Diffuse interstitial lung disease
- Endocarditis
- Glomerulonephritis
- Hemoptysis
- Hypertension
- Ischemic optic neuropathy
- Myocardial infarction
- Myocarditis
- Nasal mucosa
- Nasal polyps
- Pericarditis
- Peripheral neuropathies
- Pleural effusions
- Radiculopathies
- Renal arteritis
- Sinusitis
- Transient pulmonary infiltrates

Medical Management

Positive diagnosis is based on the presence of at least four of the following symptoms.

1. Abnormalities of paranasal sinuses
2. Bronchospasm
3. >10% eosinophil count
4. Extravascular eosinophils
5. Nonfixed pulmonary infiltrates
6. Poly- or mononeuropathy

Patients usually have a very long history of asthma. Generalized treatment of asthma is continued vigorously and must be optimized. The box below lists physiologic/anatomical abnormalities associated with Churg-Strauss syndrome.

Physiologic/Anatomical Abnormalities Associated with Churg-Strauss Syndrome

- Abnormal urine sediment, proteinuria, microscopic hematuria, and RBC casts
- Anemia
- Antineutrophil cytoplasmic antibodies (ANCA) (70% of patients are perinuclear-ANCA positive)
- Blood urea nitrogen and creatinine levels are elevated
- Elevated eosinophil cationic protein (ECP), soluble interleukin-2 receptor (sIL-2R), and soluble thrombomodulin
- Elevated IgE levels
- Eosinophilia
- Eosinophilia in bronchoalveolar lavage
- Eosinophils ≥10%
- Erythrocyte sedimentation rate and C-reactive protein level are increased
- Hypergammaglobulinemia
- Positive for rheumatoid factor at low titer

Chest X-Ray
- Hilar nodal enlargement (occasionally)
- Local parenchymal opacities
- Pulmonary opacities
- Rare cavitation
- Transient pulmonary infiltrates

Complications

If left untreated, CSS can progress to extensive cardiac involvement, which can culminate in death. Exacerbation and/or extension of the asthmatic initiating component can lead to pulmonary infiltrates and/or pleural effusions. Renal involvement can initiate hypertension or lead to its exacerbation, if already present.

Anesthesia Implications

Any surgical intervention not of an emergent nature should
be postponed, delayed, or rescheduled until the CSS treatment
is well under way and the benefits of the treatment regimen
are relatively easily observed. Before surgery and anesthesia,
treatment of the patient's asthma *must* be optimized. Pulmonary function testing is appropriate preoperatively. Cardiac,
neurologic, renal, and hepatic functions should be evaluated
preoperatively. The extent of the evaluation should be guided
by the history/progress of CSS. Enzyme induction should
be anticipated, particularly when treatment has included the
chemotherapeutic agents listed above.

Development of nasal polyps may inhibit nasal intubation,
which may be particularly important in a patient scheduled for
a maxillofacial procedure.

Pulmonary involvement can produce patches of pneumonitis, which reduces the compliance of the lungs in areas. The
reduced compliance of portions of the lungs leads to overdistention of alveoli in more compliant areas. Overdistention of
more compliant areas increases the possibility of barotraumas
during positive pressure ventilation. The development of
patches of pneumonitis also produces areas of ventilation/
perfusion mismatching and compounds any gas exchange
abnormalities already present as a result of the asthma. Therefore,
whenever possible, direct laryngoscopy, tracheal intubation,
and positive pressure ventilation are best avoided. Spontaneous
ventilation with regional anesthesia or with general anesthesia
via mask is more advantageous for the patient. The laryngeal
mask airway (LMA) may be used in appropriate surgical situations. If intubation and ventilation are unavoidable, longer
expiratory phases and/or pressure-controlled ventilatory methods should be employed to minimize the potential for alveolar
overdistention/barotrauma. Preoperative and/or intraoperative supplementation with a corticosteroid should be strongly
considered to aid with the patient's stress response.

Cor Pulmonale

Definition

Cor pulmonale is the alteration of the structure and function of the right ventricle as the result of a primary respiratory disorder. Pulmonary hypertension generally results from the connection between the primary lung dysfunction and the heart.

Incidence

Of all patients in the United States with heart disease concomitant with a form of chronic obstructive pulmonary disease (COPD), approximately 6% to 7% will develop cor pulmonale. Exact determination of the incidence of this disease is difficult since not all patients with COPD develop cor pulmonale. The incidence is heavily dependent on "local" conditions, such as local air quality, cigarette smoking, and many other lung disease risk factors.

Etiology

Numerous pathophysiologic mechanisms may produce pulmonary hypertension (see box below). Cor pulmonale is a subsequent pathophysiologic development. The involvement of the right ventricle is somewhat different, depending on whether the underlying condition is chronic or acute. In chronic cor pulmonale, the right ventricle hypertrophies over time; in an acute development situation, the right ventricle becomes dilated to the point of dysfunction.

Pathophysiologic Mechanisms Leading to Cor Pulmonale

- Idiopathic primary pulmonary hypertension
- Increased blood viscosity resulting from blood dyscrasias
- Pulmonary vascular bed compromise as the result of lung disease(s)
- Pulmonary vasoconstriction secondary to alveolar hypoxia or acidemia

---

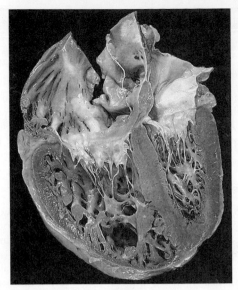

Cor Pulmonale. Chronic cor pulmonale, characterized by a markedly dilated and hypertrophied right ventricle, with thickened free wall and hypertrophied trabeculae (apical four-chamber view of heart, right ventricle on left). The shape of the left ventricle (to the right) has been distorted by the right ventricular enlargement. *(From Kumar V, Abbas AK, Fausto N: Robbins and Cotran's Pathologic Basis of Disease, ed. 7, Philadelphia, 2005, Saunders.)*

Signs and Symptoms

- Anginal chest pain
- Cough
- Dyspnea on exertion
- Fatigue
- Hemoptysis
- Hoarseness due to left recurrent laryngeal nerve compression (rare)

- Hypoxemia
- Syncope on exertion
- Tachypnea

In Advanced Disease

- Anorexia
- Passive hepatic congestion due to severe right ventricular failure
- Right upper quadrant discomfort

Medical Management

Prognosis is typically poor once cor pulmonale develops as a result of the primary pulmonary disease. The 5-year survival rate is only around 30%.

The patient with acute cor pulmonale requires intense cardiopulmonary support, including fluid loading and vasoconstrictor administration. The primary cause should be determined and corrected, to the extent possible, as soon as possible. If the cause is massive pulmonary embolism, administration of thrombolytic agents should be strongly considered and weighed against the possible need for surgical embolectomy.

Chronic cor pulmonale employs different treatments in various combinations to optimize the long-term management of the disease. The treatment options include oxygen therapy, diuretic administration, vasodilator medications, cardiac glycosides, theophylline, and anticoagulation.

Surgical intervention is indicated predominately for acute cor pulmonale. Phlebotomy may be utilized in the patient with chronic cor pulmonale and chronic hypoxia resulting in polycythemia with hematocrit values >65%. Pulmonary embolectomy has proven effective in unresolved pulmonary embolus (emboli) producing pulmonary hypertension. The patient in the terminal phase of the disease, which is further complicated by cor pulmonale, may be treated by transplantation of one lung, both lungs, or heart and lungs.

Complications

- Death
- Hypoxia
- Passive hepatic congestion
- Pedal edema
- Syncope

Anesthesia Implications

A balloon flotation pulmonary artery catheter should be an integral part of monitoring for the patient with cor pulmonale. Once placed, the device provides continuous assessment of pulmonary artery pressure, right ventricular pressure, right ventricular myocardial oxygen demand/supply balance, and pulmonary function. The pulmonary artery catheter can help distinguish between left ventricular failure and respiratory failure. Mixed venous blood sampling provides more accurate information and is a more sensitive indicator of pulmonary dysfunction than the PaO_2 values obtained from arterial blood gas analysis alone.

The degree of pulmonary hypertension has a significant impact on anesthetic management. When pulmonary hypertension is present without concomitant right ventricular failure, the patient may benefit from the use of the potent volatile inhalational anesthetic agents. High concentrations of the volatile agents may decrease hypoxic vasoconstriction and thus decrease the potential for hypoxemia.

If the patient also has pulmonary parenchymal disease and a significant bronchospastic component, incorporation of ketamine may be indicated.

Nitrous oxide may be used, but caution is highly advised because of its tendency to produce increased pulmonary artery pressure.

Hypoxia, hypercarbia, acidosis, and hypothermia should be avoided because of the predisposition to produce pulmonary vasoconstriction.

The primary objective is maintaining or preserving right ventricular function while facing the elevated right ventricular afterload. With this objective in mind, a total intravenous anesthetic technique (TIVA) utilizing an opioid (fentanyl or remifentanil) and a sedative/hypnotic (midazolam and/or propofol) may best facilitate this objective. Further concerns include ventricular preload, heart rate, and the ventricular inotropic state along with ventricular afterload.

Inotropic support is frequently necessary, particularly for the patient with cor pulmonale. The pulmonary effects of the many inotropic agents should be strongly considered before finalizing the choice for any inotropic support that may become necessary. Dobutamine and milrinone are very effective at reducing pulmonary artery pressure and pulmonary vascular resistance in patients with right ventricular failure without concomitant systemic hypotension.

Norepinephrine and epinephrine are the catecholamines of choice for cases where right ventricular contractility is significantly or severely impaired or when right ventricular perfusion pressures need to be maintained. Vasopressin is singularly effective in treating systemic hypotension in patients with right ventricular failure.

Patients may be receiving vasodilators to reduce the right ventricular afterload. These include: sodium nitroprusside, nitroglycerin, milrinone, adenosine, nifedipine, amlodipine, and prostaglandin E_1.

Nitric oxide (NO) is a selective pulmonary vascular dilator and is an effective treatment for pulmonary hypertension.

If a patient has been receiving chronic treatment with epoprostenol, inadvertent discontinuation may precipitate a *fatal* episode of pulmonary hypertension.

Cronkhite-Canada Syndrome

Definition

Cronkhite-Canada syndrome is a very rare, sporadically occurring, uninherited disorder. It is characterized by gastrointestinal polyps, cutaneous pigmentation, alopecia, and onychodystrophy.

Incidence

Cronkhite-Canada syndrome is an extremely rare disease. Since first described in 1955, 467 cases have been reported through the year 2002. The vast majority of cases have been documented in Japan, but cases have been reported world-wide. There is a very slight male to female difference in rate of incidence: 1.3:1 to 1.5:1.

The disease may manifest itself at virtually any age; however, fewer than 10 cases in infants have been reported since 1955. Cases have been reported in adults from 31 to 86 years of age.

Etiology

The etiology of Cronkhite-Canada syndrome is not known at present. Currently available evidence and data do not support a familial predisposition to developing the disease. Reports have linked incidences of the disease to arsenic poisoning.

Signs and Symptoms

- Cataracts
- Change in taste sensation
- Cheilosis papillary atrophy of the tongue
- Chronic or recurrent watery diarrhea, some-times melena
- Difficulty swallowing
- Edema (mild and peripheral to massive anasarca)
- Episodic or constant abdominal pain (upper or lower)
- Hypogeusia (may or may not be present)
- Loss of ability to smell
- Macrocephaly (infants and children)
- Muscle wasting
- Nail dystrophy leading to onycholysis

- Positive Chvostek and Trousseau signs
- Progressive anorexia
- Progressive weight loss
- Rapid alopecia (may include scalp, eyebrows, face, axillae, pubic areas, legs)
- Seizures
- Sensory neuropathy
- Skin hyperpigmentation

- Symmetric, desquamating rash on lower back, buttocks, genital areas, lips, and perioral region (infants and children)
- Syncope
- Vestibular disturbances (gaze-evoked nystagmus, disequilibrium)
- Vitiligo
- Xanthelasma

Medical Management

Therapy consists almost exclusively of interventions to treat symptoms; preventive measures are unavailable because of the lack of knowledge regarding the disease etiology. The ultimate goal is correction of fluid, electrolyte, and protein abnormalities. The patient is prone to frequent, high-volume, watery bowel movements. Regulation of the frequency of bowel movements assists in regulation of the fluid, electrolyte, and protein imbalances. Systemic corticosteroids administered in combination with an antiplasmin have demonstrated effectiveness, as have dietary changes and hyperalimentation. Antibiotics correct intestinal bacterial overgrowth. Severe anemia may necessitate transfusions.

Surgical intervention is typically reserved to treat complications of Cronkhite-Canada syndrome that may arise. These surgically amenable complications include prolapse, bowel obstruction, or malignancy.

Complications

- Cachexia
- Fluid, electrolyte, and protein imbalances
- Gastric polyp-bearing mucosal prolapse

- Gastrointestinal bleeding
- Heart failure
- Intussusception
- Thromboembolic episodes secondary to dehydration

Anesthesia Implications

The patient's fluid and electrolyte levels should be assessed preoperatively. Electrolyte imbalances should be corrected preoperatively. Protein losses and cachexia may increase the bioavailability of many anesthesia-related medications. The doses of many anesthesia-related drugs may need to be reduced because of low serum proteins and/or cachexia. Fluid level correction must be tempered to avoid heart failure, but will be helped by correction of the low serum protein levels. Chronic corticosteroid administration may require a prophylactic stress response dose of hydrocortisone. The presence of anemia may lower the transfusion threshold, particularly for larger, more complex surgical procedures.

Cystic Fibrosis

Definition

Cystic fibrosis (CF) is an ultimately lethal inherited disorder. It predominately affects the function of endocrine glands, with wide-ranging effects on multiple organ systems, including the lungs, pancreas, intestines, and liver. CF is characterized by chronic pulmonary infections and inadequate pancreatic enzymes, along with other associated complications.

Incidence

In the United States, the incidence of cystic fibrosis in Caucasians of northern European heritage is 1:3200; in the African American population, 1:15,000; in the Hispanic population, 1:9200; and in the Asian American population, 1:30,000. Internationally, the occurrence ranges from 1:620 in a specific group of Dutch heritage to 1:90,000 among Asian populations.

Etiology

Cystic fibrosis is an autosomal recessive disease, the expression of which is a defect in the gene for the cystic fibrosis transmembrane conductance regulator (CFTR). CFTR encodes a protein that is a chloride channel regulated by cyclic adenosine monophosphate (cAMP). This mutation produces cAMP-regulated chloride transport abnormalities in epithelial cells' mucosal surfaces. The subsequent chloride transport failure, along with the concomitant water transport abnormalities, culminates in very viscous secretions within the respiratory system, pancreas, gastrointestinal tract, sweat glands, and other exocrine tissues. The viscous secretions are tenacious and difficult to clear.

Lung disease is the most common reason for death among CF patients. The lungs develop quite normally in utero, are normal at birth, and for a period of time after birth. The thick, tenacious mucous secretions establish a scenario for infection that is followed by a neutrophilic inflammatory response. This cycle of infection followed by neutrophilic inflammation continues throughout the patient's life. It eventually produces structural damage, impaired gas exchange, end-stage lung disease, and finally, early death.

Signs and Symptoms

- Abdominal distention
- Cheilosis
- Cough (dry and productive)
- Cyanosis
- Digit clubbing
- Dry skin
- Hepatosplenomegaly
- Hyperresonant chest
- Increased anteroposterior chest diameter
- Kyphosis
- Nasal polyps
- Parotid gland swelling
- Rectal prolapse
- Respiratory distress
- Rhinitis
- Scoliosis
- Submandibular gland swelling
- Tachypnea
- Wheezing

Medical Management

Cystic fibrosis affects multiple organs. Management is thus a multidisciplinary effort that may involve surgery (general, cardiothoracic, or transplant), endocrinology, otolaryngology,

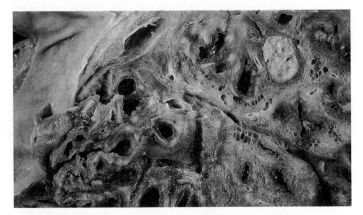

Cystic Fibrosis. This lung from a 20-year-old man shows diffuse bronchiectasis. *(From Damjanov I, Linder J:* Pathology: A Color Atlas, *St Louis, 2000, Mosby.)*

pulmonology, cardiology, and gastroenterology. Most often the patient with cystic fibrosis is treated primarily by a pulmonologist because of the prevalence of pulmonary symptoms. The viscous secretions commonly seen in the patient with cystic fibrosis create a persistent, rich growth medium for infectious organisms, such as *Haemophilus influenza*, *Klebsiella pneumoniae*, *Escherichia coli*, and *Staphylococcus aureus*. The patient typically experiences recurrent bouts of respiratory/pulmonary infections that are treated with antibiotics. They are usually very well educated about the disease, even at a young age, and receive respiratory treatments every day. One goal of the treatments is to dramatically reduce the viscosity of the secretions and facilitate expectoration of the mucus. Daily chest physiotherapy and postural drainage are often required to help facilitate expectoration of the mucus.

The patient with cystic fibrosis may be small for his or her age. The effects of this disease are far reaching. Because of the dysfunction of the pancreas caused by the disease, growth and development are impaired. Fat-soluble vitamins are not properly absorbed, which also interferes with growth and development. A high-energy, high-fat diet with fat-soluble vitamin and mineral supplementation may be required to compensate for these inadequacies. The patient with cystic fibrosis is encouraged to exercise regularly to improve physical fitness. Upper-body exercises help increase the endurance of accessory respiratory muscles.

The ultimate goals in medically managing the patient with cystic fibrosis are to: (1) maintain pulmonary function as close to normal as possible; (2) provide adequate nutrition via a high-energy, high-fat diet with supplementation of vitamins, minerals, phytonutrients, and enzymes to promote growth and development; and (3) manage any complications that develop because of the disease. As a result of advances in knowledge and understanding of cystic fibrosis, patients are living longer, more normal lives, but they still have a limited life expectancy. The most recent estimated median survival is about 30 years of age; male patients seem to survive slightly longer than female patients.

Complications

- Atelectasis
- Bronchiectasis
- Bronchiolitis
- Bronchitis
- Cholecystitis
- Chronic sinusitis

- Coagulation irregularities
- Cor pulmonale
- Cystic fibrosis–related diabetes mellitus
- Delayed puberty
- Distal intestinal obstruction syndrome
- Fatty liver
- Focal biliary cirrhosis
- Gallstones
- Gastroesophageal reflux
- Heatstroke
- Hemoptysis
- Hypertrophic pulmonary osteoarthropathy
- Liver failure
- Meconium ileus
- Mucocele
- Mucopyocele
- Nasal polyps
- Osteoporosis
- Pancreatic tissue damage
- Pneumothorax
- Portal hypertension
- Rectal prolapse
- Reduced fertility
- Rickets
- Salt depletion
- Vitamin deficiencies

Anesthesia Implications

The foremost anesthesia consideration revolves around the patient's respiratory status. The respiratory function of a patient with cystic fibrosis can deteriorate very significantly in the course of a single day. A chest x-ray should be obtained to determine whether the patient has a pneumothorax or if there are any pneumonic processes or bullous disease present.

Coagulation time should be obtained preoperatively. Determining this value gives two pieces of information. First, it reflects the patient's nutritional status—specifically, prolonged PT with normal PTT times may be the result of a vitamin K deficiency, which is a fat-soluble vitamin frequently missing from the patient's dietary intake. Second, the prolonged coagulation times alert the anesthetist to the possibility of greater-than-expected blood loss from the proposed surgical procedure. It may be necessary to administer vitamin K or fresh frozen plasma, or to consult with a hematologist to reduce the patient's possiblity of bleeding.

The effects of cystic fibrosis on the gastrointestinal tract may provoke signs and symptoms of gastroesophageal reflux disease (GERD). In such cases the patient should receive preoperative medications consistent with GERD, such as non-particulate antacids and/or H_2-receptor antagonists. Rapid sequence induction may be utilized despite the patient's higher probability for rapid desaturation when apneic.

The nature and scope of the surgical procedure proposed has considerable bearing on the anesthesia technique selected. Both general and regional techniques offer advantages. Regional anesthesia avoids manipulation of the airway, which reduces the risk of aspiration and bronchospasm. A regional technique also eliminates the requirement for positive pressure ventilation, which decreases potential for pneumothorax during the perioperative period. General anesthesia with slower respiratory rates, slightly smaller tidal volumes, humidification of inspired gases, and longer expiratory phases are beneficial because patients with cystic fibrosis are easily fatigued by the work of breathing and are capable only of marginal tidal volume exchanges on a consistent basis.

Regional anesthesia lessens the need for analgesics, particularly opioids, in the immediate postoperative period. Thus another potential source of postoperative airway compromise can be avoided.

Because of the propensity for spontaneous pneumothorax in the patient with cystic fibrosis, nitrous oxide should be avoided. Nitrous oxide can rapidly expand a pneumothorax, should one actually occur.

Cystic Hygroma

C

Definition

Cystic hygroma is a lymph angioma composed of multilocu-
lated, thin-walled cysts. It is typically benign.

Incidence

A rare congenital malformation, cystic hygroma occurs in
approximately 1:12,000 births. Because the malformation is
congenital, about 65% of the cases are obvious at birth, whereas
the remainder manifest themselves within the first 2 years of life.

Etiology

Cystic hygroma occurs as the result of a fetus's failure during
gestation to form venous drainage channels. The result is
dilated and disorganized lymph channels. The largest of these
lymph channels manifest as cystic hygromas. These cysts are
most often found in the neck (approximately 75%) with about
20% being found in the axilla. The remaining 5% may be found
virtually any place within the lymphatic system. Because of
the proximity of the lymphatic system to the neurovascular
bundles, these structures are often encompassed by the cystic
hygroma.

Signs and Symptoms

The signs and symptoms vary, depending on the location of
the lesion.
• Bluish skin discoloration over the lesion
• Cyanosis
• Soft, painless, doughy/compressible mass
• Stridor

Medical Management

The treatment of choice for cystic hygroma is surgical excision
of the hygroma. This is generally undertaken as soon as possible after the diagnosis is made.

Alternatively, sclerosing agents and/or steroids may be directly injected into the cystic hygroma. Sclerosing treatment has had variable success, particularly in view of the young age of the majority of patients with cystic hygroma, possibly as the result of the greater regenerative capabilities of younger patients.

Cystic hygromas are prone to infection. Any infection should be treated with intravenous antibiotics. Any surgical interventions that are scheduled should be postponed until the infection is resolved.

Recurrence is approximately 10%, and is more likely to occur with large cysts in the neck.

Complications

- Airway obstruction
- Deformity of the surrounding bony structures or teeth (if treatment is delayed significantly)
- Hemorrhage
- Infection

Surgical Complications
- Chylothorax
- Chylous fistula
- Hemorrhage
- Neurovascular structural damage

Anesthesia Implications

Because almost all cases of cystic hygroma occur in patients younger than 2 years of age, consideration of age-appropriate measures and developmental anxieties must be addressed. The most obvious implication, particularly in the neonate, is airway obstruction. The large size of the hygroma invades the deep fascia of the neck, oral cavity, tongue, and pharynx. As a result, oral direct laryngoscopy may be difficult, at best, and intubation may prove impossible. Nasal intubation, whether blind or using the fiberoptic bronchoscope, may be the most prudent course of action. Under the best circumstances and when fully awake, the patient with cystic hygroma may have a marginally adequate airway. This airway may be completely lost with mask induction of general anesthesia; therefore, an awake intubation may be the most appropriate intervention, especially in the very youngest patients. Despite these measures, intubation may not be possible and a surgeon *must* be readily available—in the OR suite—to perform an awake tracheostomy. The tumor may cause tracheal deviation along with other forms of encroachment.

Also, as a result of the tumor, the patient with cystic hygroma may be both malnourished and dehydrated. Despite this, an antisialagogue may be needed to reduce the copious oral secretions. On completion of the surgery and anesthesia, extremely careful consideration must be taken before extubation. It may be prudent to leave this patient intubated because of the great amount of manipulation of the tissues surrounding the airway structures and the high potential for further, continued upper airway edema.

Cystic hygromas are highly vascular and are typically found adjacent to vascular structures. One of the potential complications of surgical excision of a cystic hygroma is hemorrhage. Therefore this surgical procedure is associated with a relatively large volume of blood loss. The anesthetist must concentrate on maintaining normal volume for this patient, particularly if the patient is very young. Because of the patient's age and the relatively large volumes of fluid that may be administered, temperature shifts are also of great concern. Maintaining normothermia is thus an additional critical concern for the anesthetist.

Denervated (Transplanted) Heart

Definition

Denervated, or transplanted, heart is not a disease and is something of a misnomer. The denervated heart is a heart that has been donated and transplanted. In this case, "denervated" means the transplanted heart is not under the control of the recipient's autonomic nervous system and brain; instead, the heart rate is determined completely by the intrinsic rate(s) of the allograft heart. The atrioventricular node is predominately the rate controller for this heart because the sinus node is often irreparably damaged in the transplant process.

Incidence

About 1% of the population with end-stage congestive heart failure receive a donor heart.

Etiology

Transplants are reserved for patients with end-stage congestive heart failure who have a prognosis of less than 1 year to survive without replacement of the damaged heart.

Indications for Cardiac Transplant

- Ability to comply with follow-up care
- Age <65 years
- Congenital heart disease
- Dilated cardiomyopathy
- Ejection fraction <25%
- Intractable angina
- Ischemic cardiomyopathy
- Malignant cardiac dysrhythmias
- Pulmonary vascular resistance <2 Wood units

Contraindications to Cardiac Transplant

- Active malignancy
- Active systemic disease (collagen vascular disease, sickle-cell disease, etc.)
- Active systemic infection
- Age >65 years
- Fixed pulmonary vascular resistance >4 Wood units
- Inability to comply with follow-up care
- Ongoing history of substance abuse
- Psychosocial instability

Signs and Symptoms

Not applicable.

Medical Management

The chief concern is rejection of the transplanted heart. Various transplant centers have differing regimens of medical care for the patient with a heart transplant. These include aggressive immunosuppression (both before and after transplantation), frequent cardiac biopsies to assess for signs of organ rejection, and frequent follow-up cardiology care. Immunosuppressant levels are monitored and dosages adjusted frequently to minimize the potential for allograft rejection and to reduce the detrimental side effects of the immunosuppressants themselves.

Signs of Allograft Rejection
• Edema of extremities • Fatigue • Fever • Weight gain

Complications

- Acute rejection
- Allograft vascular disease
- Bleeding from suture lines
- Chronic rejection
- Infection
- Poor cardiac function
- Psychiatric disturbances

Anesthesia Implications

Cyclosporine is both nephro- and hepatotoxic, as well as being associated with hypertension. It is also known to lower the seizure threshold. Both renal and hepatic function should be carefully evaluated preoperatively.

Tacrolimus is also a nephrotoxic medication and has been reported to produce diabetes mellitus and hypertension.

Corticosteroid administration is associated with the development of osteoporosis and diabetes. Typically a perioperative dose of corticosteroid is needed preoperatively.

Beat-to-beat variability associated with respiratory efforts, physical activity, and vagal maneuvers is lost as a result of the transplantation process. As a result, the denervated heart will not react to the administration of atropine to treat bradycardia. Increasing the heart rate in this case will require administration of isoproterenol or by directly, artificially pacing the heart.

The denervated heart, specifically the SA and AV nodes, have been documented to be extremely sensitive to the effects of adenosine and theophylline.

Heart rate increases can be achieved by administration of catecholamines, but onset may be prolonged.

The denervated heart does not respond immediately to rapid changes in the systemic vascular resistance, as a "normal" heart would. Hypotension is poorly tolerated.

If the patient is 5 years or more post-transplantation, coronary artery disease should be given strong consideration because of the accelerated predisposition to this disease. Because of the interruption of sensory innervation during the transplantation process, the patient with a denervated heart may not experience angina in response to myocardial ischemia.

Dermatomyositis

Definition

Dermatomyositis is a disorder of collagen/connective tissue characterized by nonsuppurative skin inflammation and subcutaneous tissue and muscle fiber necrosis. It may be acute, subacute, or chronic.

Incidence

The most recent estimates indicate that dermatomyositis occurs at the rate of about 5.5:1,000,000. The frequency seems to be increasing. There is a 2:1 predilection toward females, but no apparent preference for a particular race.

Etiology

The cause of dermatomyositis is not fully understood. There are suggestions that it is caused by a complement-mediated vascular inflammation. The immunologic abnormalities may be triggered by a wide variety of agents.

Potential Triggers of Immunologic Abnormalities Related to Dermatomyositis	
• Borrelia species	• Silicone breast implants
• Collagen injections	• Toxoplasma species
• Drug ingestion	• Viruses

Signs and Symptoms

- Arthralgia
- Arthritis
- Calcinosis of skin or muscle
- Dysphagia
- Dysphonia
- Dyspnea
- Dysrhythmias
- Facial erythema
- Gottron papules
- Heliotrope rash
- Joint swelling
- Malar erythema
- Muscle tenderness
- Muscle weakness
- Poikiloderma
- Pruritic skin lesions
- Psoriasis from dermatitis

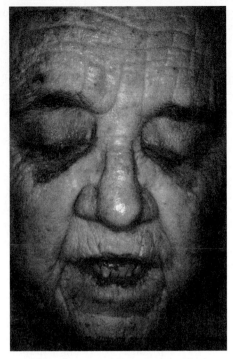

Dermatomyositis. Note the rash affecting the eyelids. *(From Kumar V, Abbas AK, Fausto N: Robbins and Cotran's Pathologic Basis of Disease, ed. 7, Philadelphia, 2005, Saunders.)*

Medical Management

The muscle inflammation discomfort benefits from inactivity, such as bed rest. Physical therapy, on the other hand, helps counteract the muscle weakness and helps prevent contractures.

Some patients develop dysphagia and may be more prone to aspiration and aspiration pneumonia; the occurrence of both can be reduced by avoiding eating for several hours before bedtime. The incidence of reflux/aspiration can also be decreased by elevating the head of the bed.

Aside from bed rest and physical therapy, systemic corticosteroids are a standard of treatment. Prednisone is the typical first-line drug used. On establishing remission, the drug is tapered to discontinuation over time to reduce the probability of a relapse.

Chronic administration of corticosteroids often results in the development of toxic effects. These effects are frequently counteracted by initiation of an immunosuppressive or cytotoxic drug. Methotrexate is usually the drug of choice for the steroid-sparing medication; however, azathioprine and mycophenolate mofetil are viable alternatives. Intravenous administration of high-dose immunoglobulin is reserved for the patient for whom steroids and/or immunosuppressant/cytotoxic therapy proves unsuccessful. It is carried out monthly, and generally produces only short-term benefits.

The cutaneous aspects of this disease are the most difficult to treat. The first-line intervention is for the patient to realize and understand the photosensitive nature of the disease. The patient should limit exposure to the sun as much as possible, either by outright avoidance or by application of copious amounts of sunscreen solution. Other practical actions include wearing broad-brimmed hats, using umbrellas, and covering skin with clothing. There have been reports of beneficial effects of hydroxychloroquine and chloroquine on the cutaneous manifestations of this disease.

Calcinosis is debilitating if it becomes established. Remission is possible, but if it occurs, it is only after the patient has had the disease for years. This complication has reportly been gradually resolved by administration of the calcium channel–blocking drug, diltiazem.

Complications

- Aspiration
- Aspiration pneumonia
- Calcinosis
- Cardiac conduction abnormalities
- Congestive heart failure
- Contractures
- Dysphagia
- Gastrointestinal ulcers and perforations
- Interstitial lung disease
- Myocarditis
- Necrotizing vasculitis

Anesthesia Implications

Dysphagia increases the potential for aspiration, particularly during induction of general anesthesia. Prudence dictates that the patient receive a rapid sequence induction.

Muscle weakness is a hallmark of this disease. It is especially evident in the neck flexors and shoulder and pelvic girdles. Administration of muscle relaxants may need to be reduced because these muscle groups exhibit greater sensitivity to them. On completion of anesthesia, even though reversal is deemed complete, the patient may not be able to produce a sustained head-lift because of the already weak neck muscles.

Interstitial lung disease may proceed to restrictive lung disease. As a result, diffusing capacity is diminished and the potential for air trapping increases, as does the potential for barotrauma. When positive pressure ventilation is required, peak inspiratory pressures should be reduced while expiratory time is increased to reduce the potential for lung injury.

The patient's respiratory capabilities should be thoroughly assessed preoperatively utilizing pulmonary function testing, in particular vital capacity, arterial blood gas analysis, and chest x-rays. If the patient's capabilities are deemed marginal, the patient should not be allowed to spontaneously breathe either intra- or postoperatively. In such cases general anesthesia would be the more appropriate choice for anesthesia technique. Regional anesthesia should be used in combination with general anesthesia. Postoperative mechanical ventilatory should be anticipated for the patient with dermatomyositis who receives general anesthesia.

Cardiac conduction abnormalities increase the potential for development of detrimental dysrhythmias.

Chronic administration of corticosteroids requires a perioperative dose of steroid before surgical incision.

Renal function should be assessed preoperatively. The patient with dermatomyositis may develop necrotizing vasculitis, which may affect renal function.

DiGeorge Syndrome

Definition

DiGeorge syndrome is a congenital disorder involving hypoplasia or aplasia of the thymus and parathyroid glands secondary to defective development of the third and fourth pharyngeal pouches.

Incidence

DiGeorge syndrome occurs very sporadically. The prevalence is the subject of much debate; however, current estimates of the incidence range from 1:4000 to 1:6395. Male to female ratio is 1:1.

Etiology

The anomaly results from deletion of the DiGeorge syndrome chromosome region (DGCR), represented as deletion on chromosome 22q11.2.

Conditions Associated with DiGeorge Syndrome

- 22q11 deletion syndromes
- Cayler syndrome*
- CHARGE syndrome (see box)
- Conotruncal anomaly face syndrome*
- Opitz-GBBB syndrome*
- Velocardiofacial syndrome

*See Appendix G: Rare Syndroms.

CHARGE Association

Coloboma of the iris, choroid, and/or microphthalmia
Heart defect
Atresia of the choanae
Retarded growth and development
Genitourinary abnormalities (cryptorchidism, microphallus, hydronephrosis)
Ear defects associated with deafness

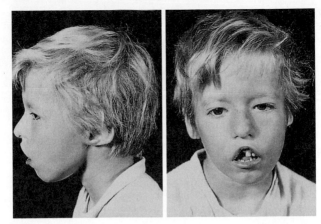

DiGeorge Syndrome. Facial anomalies associated with DiGeorge syndrome. Note the wide-set eyes, low-set ears, and shortened structure of the upper lip. *(From Roitt I, Brostoff J, Male D: Immunology, ed. 6, St Louis, 2001, Mosby.)*

Signs and Symptoms

Cardiac
- Aberrant right subclavian artery
- Right aortic arch
- Tetralogy of Fallot
- Truncus arteriosus
- Type B aortic arch interruption

Facial
- Bulbous nose with square tip
- Choanal atresia
- Cleft lip (rare)
- Cleft palate
- Downward slanting eyes
- Hypernasal voice
- Hypertelorism
- Low-set ears with deficient vertical diameter
- Micrognathia
- Short philtrum
- Small mouth
- Telecanthus with short palpebral fissures
- Upward slanting eyes

Gastrointestinal
- Esophageal atresia
- Imperforate anus
- Intestinal malrotation
- Tracheoesophageal (TE) fistula

Genitourinary
- Renal cystic dysplasia
- Ureterohydronephrosis

Immunologic
- Frequent infections
- Immunodeficiencies

Intellectual/Psychiatric
- Affective disorders
- Major depressive disorders
- Mental retardation
- Mild-to-moderate learning difficulties
- Paranoid schizophrenia

Nervous System
- Holoprosencephaly
- Hydrocephalus
- Meningocele
- Neural crest disturbances

Skeletal
- Short stature

Medical Management

DiGeorge syndrome is characterized by hypoparathyroidism and hypocalcemia. Both of these can be effectively treated by administration of calcium supplements as well as vitamin D.

The hypoplastic or aplastic thymus results in immunodeficiency. The deficiencies in T-cells and/or B-cells may be treated with standard prophylactic regimens. Early thymus transplantation may hasten recovery of immune function.

There are numerous clinical features of DiGeorge syndrome (see Signs and Symptoms). Many of these associated features can be rectified surgically, particularly the cardiac anomalies, such as tetralogy of Fallot or truncus arteriosus.

Complications

- Cardiac dysrhythmias secondary to hypocalcemia
- Immunodeficiency
- Recurrent infections

Anesthesia Implications

Securing the airway of the patient with DiGeorge syndrome may be difficult. The patient typically has micrognathia and a small mouth, both of which contribute to making direct laryngoscopy difficult. Direct glottis visualization may prove impossible. It may be necessary to use the laryngeal mask airway (LMA) where appropriate for the proposed surgical procedure. For more complex surgical procedures, the intubating LMA may be required. It may be necessary to use the fiberoptic bronchoscope for intubating purposes. Because the patient may have choanal atresia, the nasal route for intubation may not be available, leaving only the oral route for intubation purposes. The difficult airway cart must be immediately at hand, and a surgeon should be available to surgically secure the airway if necessary.

The hypocalcemia associated with DiGeorge syndrome can affect the delivery of anesthesia. The patient's response to neuromuscular blocking drugs may be significantly altered. Acute hypocalcemia secondary to hypoparathyroidism can contribute to hemodynamic instability. Hypocalcemia may be exacerbated by hyperventilation and the resultant respiratory alkalosis. The worsening hypocalcemia may further affect response to neuromuscular blockade.

The patient with DiGeorge syndrome is prone to develop infections because the hypoplastic or aplastic thymus gland suppresses cell-mediated immunity.

Hypocalcemia can delay ventricular repolarization, resulting in a prolonged Q-T interval. As a result, the patient may develop a 2:1 heart block. Hypocalcemia may culminate in seizures, which can be exacerbated by the administration of anticonvulsants.

Duchenne's Dystrophy

Definition

Duchenne's dystrophy is a chronic, progressive, severe pseudohypertrophic muscular dystrophy—the most commonly occurring type. It is characterized by increasing weakness of pelvic and shoulder girdle musculature, pseudohypertrophy of the muscles, then atrophy and lordosis. People with the disease have a peculiar, particular swinging gait (waddling gait) with the legs kept wide apart.

Diagnostic Criteria for Duchenne's Dystrophy

- Absence of bowel or bladder dysfunction
- Hyperlordosis with wide-based gait
- Hypertrophy of weak muscles
- Progressive course over time
- Reduced muscle contractility and electrical stimulation in advanced disease
- Sensory distribution or febrile illness
- Weakness, with onset in the legs

Signs and Symptoms of Rhabdomyolysis

- Hyperphosphatemia
- Hyperuricemia
- Lactic acidosis
- Loss of P wave or sine wave
- Peaked T waves
- Prolonged P-R and QRS intervals
- Rising creatinine phosphokinase levels
- Severe hyperkalemia
- Tea-colored urine

Incidence

This form of muscular dystrophy occurs at the rate of 1:3300 to 1:3500 births, and affects males much more often than females.

Etiology

Duchene's dystrophy is the result of a sex-linked, recessive inheritance. A mutation in the dystrophin gene is found on

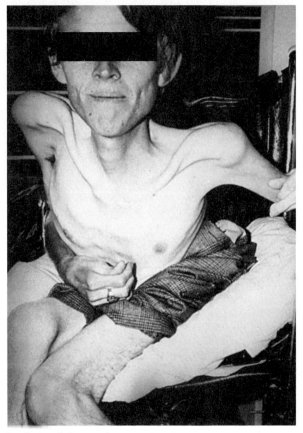

Duchenne's Dystrophy. An individual with late-stage Duchenne muscular dystrophy, showing severe muscle loss. *(From Jorde LB, et al: Medical Genetics [updated for 2006-2007], ed. 3, St Louis, 2006, Mosby.)*

the X-chromosome at the Xp21 stripe. The resultant loss of dystrophin is the first step in an interdependent series of events that includes the loss of other portions of the dystrophin-associated glycoprotein complex, breakdown of the sarcolemma with influx of calcium ions, phospholipase activation, and oxidative cellular injury. The process culminates in myonecrosis. With progression of the myonecrosis, and thus the disease, dead muscle fibers are removed by macrophages. The subsequent void is filled by both fatty and connective tissue to such an extent that the muscle appears to grow and is deceptively healthy in outward appearance, which accounts for the pseudo-hypertrophy.

Signs and Symptoms

- Atelectasis development
- Calf muscle pseudohyper-trophy
- Contractures of iliotibial bands, hip flexors, and heel cords
- Episodes of pneumonia
- Gower sign (child that pushes on knees to stand up)
- Gradual, progressive diminution of deep tendon reflexes until they disappear completely
- Kyphoscoliosis
- Signs of nocturnal hypoxemia (lethargy, early morning headache)
- Waggling gait (particularly 3- to 6-year-old boys)
- Waning forced vital capacity

Medical Management

Duchenne's dystrophy remains an incurable disease. Its symptoms can be treated and the progression retarded, but it cannot be reversed. Prednisone is the only medication that produces any benefits that modify the progression of the disease. The muscle wasting that is so debilitating can be retarded by administration of prednisone at 0.05 to 0.75 mg/kg/day in divided doses on alternating days. Benefits from treatment with prednisone may become clinically evident within a month of initiation of the treatment. The observed benefit may last as long as 3 years.

The remainder of the medical management of Duchenne's dystrophy is geared toward managing symptoms and delaying the inevitable for as long as possible. Daily exercises of joints and muscle stretching delay the onset of contractures. The stretching exercises are combined with judicious application of braces, such as foot/ankle or knee/ankle/foot orthoses, to work synergistically to help the patient maintain the ability to stand, whether mobile or not, and delay the onset of contractures and scoliosis. The onset of wheelchair dependency initiates the development of greater debilities, such as contractures, scoliosis, and degradation of muscle strength. These debilities contribute to pulmonary function impairment and gastrointestinal dysmotility.

Confinement to a wheelchair hastens, somewhat, the development of Duchenne's dystrophy. Onset of the sedentary life of muscle weakness contributes to the manifestation of complications associated with the disease. Chronic steroid use weakens the skin, making it friable and highly susceptible to breakdown and ulceration. The skin breakdown and ulceration dramatically increases the potential for infection and sepsis. Progression of the muscle weakness reduces pulmonary function. Scoliosis and hyperlordosis, the result of contractures within the spinal column, lead to development of restrictive pulmonary disease. Loss of function of the accessory muscles of breathing, the intercostals, and sternocleidomastoids contributes further to the loss of pulmonary function and the possible development of atelectasis and pneumonia. Continuous positive airway pressure (CPAP) or bi-level positive airway pressure (BiPAP) are two minimally invasive methods of pulmonary support. Development of atelectasis and pneumonia can be thwarted by frequent daily use of incentive spirometry. Broad-spectrum antibiotics may be required if pneumonia does develop. As the disease progresses, pulmonary function continues to decline, often producing increasing restrictions and ultimately creating the necessity for a tracheostomy to reduce some of the work of breathing.

Dystrophin is also found significantly in cardiac and brain tissues. As such, loss of dystrophin in these two tissues produces cardiac dysfunction and mental developmental delays. Pseudohypertrophy may also occur in the heart leading to cardiac fibrosis. Cardiac fibrosis, in turn, results in reduced cardiac output with ensuing pulmonary congestion that spirals down to fulminate congestive heart failure. The cardiac fibrosis also affects the cardiac conduction system, which may be evidenced by tall R waves in the V_1 lead, deep Q waves in the AVL, AVR, and AVF leads, shortened PR interval, and sinus tachycardia. Lethal dysrhythmias may occur.

Loss of dystrophin from cerebral tissue leads to developmental delays and diminished intellectual development. There is a shift to the left with regard to intelligence quotient (IQ) distribution, with a mean IQ being about 83 for these patients.

Complications

See Becker's dystrophy (p. 45).

Anesthesia Implications

- Atelectasis
- Cardiac conduction abnormalities
- Cardiac fibrosis
- Congestive heart failure
- Contractures
- Cushingoid habitus
- Developmental delays
- Diminished intellectual development
- Gastric ulcers
- Infection
- Muscle atrophy
- Muscle weakness
- Pneumonia
- Pressure sores
- Sepsis
- Weight gain

Eaton-Lambert Myasthenic Syndrome

E

Definition

Eaton-Lambert myasthenic syndrome (ELMS) is an autoimmune disease in which autoantibodies attack the voltage-gated calcium channels (VGCC), thus interfering with the release of acetylcholine at the presynaptic motor nerve terminal. Eaton-Lambert myasthenic syndrome is also known as Lambert-Eaton myasthenic syndrome.

Incidence

The most recent "best" estimate for the occurrence of ELMS is 1:100,000.

Etiology

Patients diagnosed with ELMS usually have some form of cancer, whether or not it has been diagnosed. Clinical manifestations of ELMS typically precede the identification of the form of cancer present. Usually, the cancer is identified within 2 years of the ELMS diagnosis. Evidence accumulating over recent years indicates that active zone particles (AZPs) represent the VGCC and align in regular parallel arrays along the presynaptic muscle membrane. In ELMS patients, divalent antibodies act on the VGCCs, cross-linking these gates and causing disruption of the parallel arrays. This disruption causes AZPs to cluster and ultimately decrease. The process culminates in the characteristic weakness of this disorder.

Carcinomas Associated with Eaton-Lambert Myasthenic Syndrome	
• Bladder carcinoma	• Lymphosarcoma
• Breast carcinoma	• Malignant thymoma
• Colon carcinoma	• Prostate carcinoma
• Gallbladder carcinoma	• Small-cell lung cancer
• Kidney carcinoma	• Stomach carcinoma

Signs and Symptoms

- Difficulty chewing
- Difficulty raising the arms
- Diminished or absent deep tendon reflexes
- Diplopia
- Dry eyes
- Dry mouth
- Dry skin
- Dysarthria
- Dysphagia
- Impotence
- Metallic taste
- Myalgia
- Postural hypotension
- Progressive weakness of proximal muscles (especially lower extremities)
- Ptosis
- Waddling gait

Medical Management

Once the diagnosis of ELMS is confirmed, the next action must be an almost exhaustive battery of testing to determine the existence of some form of malignancy. If a malignancy is discovered, the focus of treatment is to eradicate it, which by extension often results in improvement of the weakness of ELMS. If no malignancy is uncovered, the focus should shift to a relatively aggressive immunotherapy to bring about ELMS improvement.

Pharmacologic treatment of ELMS alone is focused on administration of medications that result in increased acetylcholine (ACh) transmission across the neuromuscular junction. The increased ACh transmission can occur as a primary action or a secondary result. The increased transmission can be brought about primarily with a medication that causes increased ACh release at the neuromuscular junction; increased transmission may occur secondarily with a medication that decreases the action of acetylcholinesterase.

If weakness persists, the next step is initiation of aggressive immunotherapy. Either plasma exchange (PX) or high-dose intravenous immunoglobulin gamma (IVIgG) may be utilized first because of the rapid improvement each produces. However, the resultant improvements are short lived. More long-lasting benefits may be achieved by initiation of immunosuppression therapy, most often with prednisone and azathioprine or cyclosporine either singularly or in combination.

Progression of ELMS is predicated on the presence or absence of an underlying malignancy along with the presence and severity of associated autoimmune disease. The severity and distribution of muscular weakness affects the prognosis of the patient as well. Since ELMS almost always leads to discovery of an underlying malignancy, its detection leads to earlier treatment for the resulting malignancy, which improves survival potential.

Complications

Most complications are associated with the therapies used to treat ELMS. Other complications include:

- Ataxia
- Autonomic instability
- Bleeding
- Bone marrow depression
- Cardiac dysrhythmias
- Clotting factors depletion
- Cough
- Diarrhea
- Hypercalcemia
- Insomnia
- Liver failure
- Palpitations
- Peripheral paresthesias
- Renal tubular necrosis
- Seizures

Anesthesia Implications

Patients being treated with guanidine hydrochloride should have preoperative liver function tests, a 12-lead electrocardiogram, and renal function assessment. Each of these organs can be greatly affected by guanidine.

ELMS patients are more sensitive to both depolarizing and nondepolarizing muscle relaxants. ELMS patients being treated with pyridostigmine and 3,4-diaminopyridine (DAP) may not be amenable to antagonism of muscle relaxants at the end of surgery.

ELMS patients have reduced respiratory reserves due to the muscle weakness. As a result, these patients are at greater risk for respiratory failure even with minimal exposure to volatile anesthetics and/or sedation.

Patients receiving prednisone should receive a perioperative dose of hydrocortisone because of the adrenal suppression long-term use of corticosteroids may produce.

For patients who have required multiple plasma exchanges, blood loss may be disproportionate to the surgical procedure. Bleeding times should be evaluated preoperatively. If these times are excessive, elective surgery should be postponed until therapeutic measures can bring about some correction of clotting factors and bring the bleeding times closer to normal.

Ehlers-Danlos Syndrome

Definition

Ehlers-Danlos syndrome (EDS) is a group of inherited connective tissue disorders that vary according to clinical and biochemical evidence, inheritance mode, and disorder severity (mild to lethal). The disorder is characterized by joint hyperextension, skin hyperextensibility, easy bruising, tissue friability, bleeding, poor wound healing, subcutaneous nodules, as well as cardiovascular, orthopedic, intestinal, and ocular defects.

Incidence

There are six types of Ehlers-Danlos syndrome (see table). The frequency of all recognized types of EDS is not exactly known but is estimated to be 1:5000 to 10,000. There is no discernable racial predilection.

Six Types of Ehlers-Danlos Syndrome	
Type	**Major Characteristic(s)**
Classic	Skin hyperextensibility; wide atrophic scars; joint hypermobility
Hypermobility	Joint hypermobility; soft, smooth, velvety skin
Vascular	Arterial/intestinal fragility or rupture; extensive bleeding; thin, translucent skin
Kyphoscoliosis	Joint laxity; severe neonatal hypotonia; scoliosis; progressive scleral fragility or globe rupture
Arthrochalasia	Congenital bilateral hip dislocations; severe joint hypermobility; recurrent subluxations
Dermatosparaxis	Severe skin fragility; saggy, redundant skin

Etiology

Ehlers-Danlos syndrome is an autosomal inherited disorder. The type of EDS the patient has differs according to the chromosome locus/loci and specific gene(s) abnormality.

Causes of Ehlers-Danlos Syndrome

Type of EDS	Chromosome Locus (Loci)	Gene(s) Abnormality
Classic	9q34.2-34.3; 2q31	COL5A1; COL5A2
Hypermobility	Unknown	Unknown
Vascular	2q31	COL3A1
Kyphoscoliosis	1p36.3-36.2	PLOD1
Arthrochalasia	17q31-22.5; 7q22.1	COL1A1; COL1A2
Dermatosparaxis	5q23-24	ADAMST2

Signs and Symptoms

The following signs and symptoms are common to all EDS types:

- Alveolar bone loss
- Bladder diverticula or rupture
- Bony dysplasias
- Easy bruising
- Excessive joint dislocations
- Joint hypermobility
- Microcornea
- Micrognathia
- Mitral valve prolapse
- Myopia
- Occipital exostoses
- Periodontitis
- Poor wound healing
- Prominent venous markings
- Retinal detachment
- Scoliosis
- Short stature
- Skin hyperextensibility
- Spontaneous medium-sized artery rupture
- Spontaneous viscus rupture(s)
- Tissue fragility
- Wide/thin scars

Medical Management

The first, most critical step is correctly diagnosing the syndrome. Because this disorder family affects connective tissues, careful, thorough cardiac evaluation is essential. Mitral valve prolapse is particularly common in EDS patients and should be carefully described and confirmed using an echocardiogram. Frequent, serial cardiovascular evaluations are particularly important for vascular EDS patients because of the higher risk of aneurysm formation and rupture.

Patients should be closely monitored for development and progression of scoliosis. Patients with scoliosis should be cautioned to minimize activities that produce excessive stress and strain to their back because of the hypermobility of their joints.

Lacerations and similar injuries should be carefully tended. The patient's tissue friability and fragility, as well as the wide

Ehlers-Danlos Syndrome. A, Hyperextensible joint seen in Ehlers-Danlos
syndrome. **B,** Skin laxity in Ehlers-Danlos syndrome. *(From Graham-Brown R,
Bourke J: Mosby's Color Atlas and Text of Dermatology, ed. 2, Edinburgh, 2007,
Mosby.)*

scarring associated with the disorder, are a contraindication for
use of sutures for wound closure. Better alternatives for wound
closure in the EDS patient include wound/tissue glue and/or
adhesive strips.

Complications

- Bowel perforation
- Death
- Detached retina
- Hollow viscus perforation
  or rupture
- Pneumothorax
- Spontaneous arterial
  rupture
- Uncontrollable
  hemorrhage
- Wound dehiscence

Anesthesia Implications

Correctly positioning a patient with EDS is critical. The hyper-mobility of the joints predisposes the patient to joint injuries, particularly during emergence from anesthesia. The anesthetist must also take great care to secure the patient's extremities to armboards or tuck them at the patient's side while using copious padding to minimize or prevent pressure/compression injury, such as bruising.

The tissue fragility, poor wound healing, scarring, bruising, and propensity for bleeding present something of a quandary to the anesthetist. Intramuscular injections should be avoided, if possible, making adequate anxiolysis difficult. Obtaining intra-venous access on the first attempt (ideal for any patient) takes on added importance for the EDS patient. A central venous catheter must be placed with great caution because of the increased risk of pneumothorax, as well as the greater potential for extensive hematoma formation. The increased potential for extensive hematoma formation must be factored into the deci-sion for placement of an intra-arterial catheter. Once any of these invasive lines has been inserted, methods to secure those lines must be carefully considered. Tape applied to the skin should be minimized, and gauze wrap should be used whenever possible. In addition, the intravenous and intra-arterial lines must be inspected frequently to prevent or at least minimize extravasation of fluids, which can be extensive because of the hyperextensibil-ity of the patient's skin. This measure is of increased importance to the anesthetist because of the tissue damage that can occur with extravasation of any number of anesthesia-related drugs.

The anesthetist must be even more cautious than usual during direct laryngoscopy to minimize trauma to the tissues because of increased potential for bleeding and bruising. Because of the increased potential for pneumothorax, assisted and controlled ventilation can be injurious to the patient with EDS. The anesthetist should choose the pressure-controlled ventilation option that is available on most newer anesthesia machines and opt for the lowest appropriate inspiratory pressure possible to maintain adequate ventilation and gas exchange. The expiratory phase for the patient with EDS should also be prolonged, to as much as 1:2.5 or 1:3, to reduce the possibil-ity of air trapping and barotrauma. Surgical wound dehiscence is another possible complication for the patient with EDS. The anesthetist can help reduce the potential for dehiscence by extubating the patient while relatively deeply anesthetized or by continuing mechanical ventilation and muscle paralysis into the post-anesthesia care unit.

Regional anesthesia for the patient with EDS is relatively contraindicated because of the higher potential for bleeding and extensive hematoma formation. For this same cause, the anesthetist should anticipate greater-than-normal blood volume losses for a given surgical intervention. As a result, it may be prudent to obtain blood type and antibody screening preoperatively, in the event transfusion becomes necessary during the course of surgery.

E

Eisenmenger Syndrome

Definition

Eisenmenger syndrome (ES) is the presence of a bidirectional or exclusively right-to-left cardiac shunt in conjunction with pulmonary hypertension and a patent heart defect.

Incidence

Congenital heart defects occur in approximately 1% of all live births. Out of this group, approximately 8% overall, and 11% of those with a left-to-right shunt, will eventually develop ES.

Etiology

ES is a rare disorder that affects both the respiratory and cardiac systems. This disorder is very insidious and sinister. Fulminate signs and symptoms of the disorder do not typically manifest until the third, fourth, or fifth decade of life.

The patient with ES has a congenital heart defect that has never been surgically repaired; for example, an atrial or ventricular septal defect. The blood shunted from the left side of the heart through the right side increases the stroke volume of the right side of the heart. The increased stroke volume produces shear forces within the pulmonary microvasculature. The shear forces combine with the increased stroke volume to produce irreversible damage to the walls of the pulmonary vessels. The damage to these vessel walls scars the vessels, making them less compliant.

Eventually the pulmonary vascular resistance (PVR) becomes equal to and finally exceeds the systemic vascular resistance (SVR). The shunt becomes bidirectional and eventually reverses to an exclusively right-to-left shunt, mixing deoxygenated blood with oxygenated blood, resulting in chronic hypoxemia.

Signs and Symptoms

- Angina
- Clubbing of digits
- Cyanosis
- Dyspnea on exertion
- Fatigue
- Hemoptysis
- Palpitations
- Polycythemia
- Syncope

Medical Management

The primary focus of current medical management of ES is on reducing the PVR and, by extension, the right-to-left shunting and cyanosis. Medications and treatments that have detrimental effects must be avoided. For example, calcium channel–blocking agents must be avoided; even though these medications produce reductions in the PVR, they also produce unacceptably greater reductions in the SVR, effectively exacerbating the right-to-left shunting.

Sildenafil and L-arginine are effective in decreasing or reducing the degree of pulmonary hypertension. L-Arginine is converted to nitric oxide (NO) *in vivo*, which activates guanylate cyclase. Guanylate cyclase increases the level of cyclic guanosine monophosphate (cGMP), which is instrumental in relaxing the smooth muscles of the pulmonary blood vessels. Sildenafil inhibits the degradation of cGMP, thus fostering greater cGMP availability. Sildenafil works synergistically with inhaled NO to enhance the effects of both in the NO-cGMP pathway. Combining sildenafil with L-arginine enhances the NO-cGMP pathway in an effort to effectively reduce the PVR.

Two other medications are used to treat ES patients: epoprostenol and bosentan. Epoprostenol is a prostacyclin analogue that has two primary pharmacologic actions: direct vasodilation of pulmonary and systemic vascular beds and inhibition of platelet aggregation. It also contributes to bronchodilation. This medication must be administered via a permanent central venous access.

Bosentan is an endothelin antagonist. It binds two endothelin-1 receptors, ET_A and ET_B, found in the endothelium and vascular smooth muscles. By binding to both receptors, the PVR may be reduced by as much as 25%. This reduction in the PVR by bosentan improves both the functional status and oxygenation of the patient with ES.

Finally, the patient with ES eventually develops polycythemia in an effort to counteract the chronic hypoxemia from the right-to-left shunt. Hematocrit values of 60% to 75% are not unheard of with these patients. The patient who manifests symptoms such as headaches, hemoptysis, or increased dyspnea, is treated by therapeutic phlebotomy. The phlebotomy must be carefully and strictly controlled and must be accompanied by a careful equal-volume fluid replacement of the blood that is removed in order to avoid decreasing the SVR and exacerbating the right-to-left shunt. The goal of the therapeutic phlebotomy is to reduce the red cell mass and viscosity of the blood while maintaining the SVR throughout the procedure. Therapeutic phlebotomy typically consists of removing approximately 500 mL of blood with volume-for-volume replacement with salt-free albumin, fresh frozen plasma, dextran, or isotonic saline.

Complications

- Azotemia
- Cerebrovascular accident (CVA)
- Cholelithiasis
- Decreased glomerular filtration rate
- Gout
- Hemoptysis
- Hypertrophic osteoarthropathy
- Nephrotic syndrome
- Polycythemia
- Pulmonary vasculature friability
- Renal dysfunction
- Sudden death

Anesthesia Implications

The patient with ES presents a unique challenge. The right-to-left shunt already present is easily exacerbated. This patient is very sick, often debilitated. The patient with ES is typically very anxious when faced with the possibility of surgery and anesthesia. The initial step in relieving at least a part of this anxiety is the appearance of a poised, calm, unhurried anesthesia professional equipped and ready to deal with any situation that may be presented. The attempt to obtain intravenous access will be closely scrutinized by the patient as well as family member(s). It is critically important that *all* air must be flushed from the administration tubing with the same degree of care and concern that would be given to the IV access of a neonate. Even the smallest air bubble within the pulmonary microvasculature of the patient with ES may become a significant embolism. The chief anesthetic concern mirrors the chief concern in the medical management of ES: avoiding worsening of the right-to-left shunt. The anesthetist must strive to minimize, if not avoid outright, decreases in the SVR. Whether regional or general anesthesia is the technique chosen, very nearly every anesthesia medication—inhaled vola-tiles, intravenous, or local anesthetics—may result in decreases in the patient's SVR.

Induction of general anesthesia can best be achieved using ketamine rather than thiopental, propofol, or etomi-date, which result in unacceptably large drops in the SVR. Intubation can be facilitated using a nondepolarizing muscle relaxant (NDMR). However, if the patient is receiving epoprostenol and/or bosentan, metabolism of steroid-based NDMRs, such as rocuronium, may be prolonged. The newest volatile agents, desflurane and sevoflurane, are the more appropriate choice because of the rapidity with which the depth of anesthesia can be altered with either agent. Of these two agents, desflurane may be more supportive of the SVR because of the mild sympathetic stimulation it can produce.

The goal of mechanical ventilation with the patient with ES is more to reduce the carbon dioxide (CO_2) concentration than to increase levels of oxygen saturation. Elevated CO_2 concentration results in acidosis, which increases the PVR and exacerbates the right-to-left shunting.

Pain control is vitally important for the patient with ES, both perioperatively and postoperatively. Pain produces increas-es in PVR, SVR, and cardiac oxygen requirements. Changes in any one of these parameters may be greatly magnified in the patient with ES.

An alternative to general anesthesia is total intravenous anesthesia (TIVA). Induction with ketamine remains the best choice and may be accompanied by a remifentanil infusion. Direct laryngoscopy should be facilitated using an NDMR as described earlier. After induction and intubation, an infusion of propofol may be initiated. The infusion rate should be based on, and adjusted by, the patient's blood pressure and the method of awareness monitoring of the anesthetist's or facility's choice.

Regional anesthesia is a viable alternative to general anesthe-sia. Once again, the greatest concern centers on maintaining the SVR at levels as nearly normal as possible. Adequate fluid loading before instillation of the regional anesthetic is vitally important. Epidural anesthesia or continuous subarachnoid infusion are both effective. Both are superior to the usual single-injection method of subarachnoid blockade. Both con-tinuous subarachnoid infusion and epidural anesthesia allow the onset and level of the blockade to be adjusted more gradually, which allows the patient to adjust physiologically and the anesthetist to aid that adjustment by administering additional fluids and/or appropriate vasoactive medication as needed.

Patient monitoring is necessarily more extensive with the patient with ES. Central venous pressure (CVP) and radial artery blood pressure monitoring are integral parameters for estimating the patient's SVR and PVR. Pulmonary artery balloon flotation catheter use is somewhat controversial owing to the potential difficulty in achieving proper terminal positioning and the inconsistent measurements that may be obtained from dilated, relatively noncompliant pulmonary vessels. Transesophageal echocardiography is particularly pertinent in the patient with ES undergoing large and/or lengthy surgical procedures, where greater fluid shifts and/or administrations are anticipated. Also, owing to the precarious fluid balance of the patient with ES, the period without oral intake, particularly

Patent congenital heart defect

↓

Left-to-right shunt

↓

Increased right heart stroke volume + Shearing forces

↓

Irreversible pulmonary vascular injury

↓

Increased PVR

↓

Bidirectional and/or exclusive right-to-left shunting

↓

Hypoxemia, polycythemia

Pathophysiology of Eisenmenger Syndrome.

clear liquids, should be limited—possibly to no more than 4 hours. Once again, the careful approach is similar to that taken with a neonate being prepared for surgery.

Finally, blood loss is always a concern for the anesthetist. In the patient with ES, surgical blood loss must be strictly assessed. The blood lost in the surgical field must be treated as if the patient is undergoing a therapeutic phlebotomy; that is, blood must be replaced volume-for-volume with one of the appropriate solutions noted earlier. The anesthetist must be vigilant and act quickly in anticipation because the blood lost from the surgical field does not occur in the relatively controlled manner of a therapeutic phlebotomy.

Encephalocele

Definition

Encephalocele is a herniation of a portion of the brain and/or meninges through a defect of the bony skull table. The condition may be congenital or result from trauma or surgery.

Incidence

In the United States the incidence is 1 to 4:10,000 live births; internationally there is no estimate available. Females are affected more often than males.

Etiology

Congenital encephalocele is produced by a defect in the closure of the embryonic neural tube. The closure defect results in an abnormality of the skull and meninges. Encephalocele may also occur as the result of failed basilar ossification. This defect can potentially occur at several skull locations.

Anomalies Associated with Encephalocele

- Arnold-Chiari II malformation
- Brain migrational anomalies
- Chemke syndrome*
- Corpus callosum agenesis
- Cryptophthalmos syndrome
- Dandy-Walker malformation*
- Knobloch syndrome
- Meckel-Gruber syndrome*
- Roberts syndrome*
- Spina bifida
- Trisomy 18
- von Voss syndrome*

*See Appendix G: Rare Syndromes.

Locations and Frequencies of Encephalocele

Bony Defect	Occurrence Percentage
Occipital	75%
Frontoethmoidal	13% to 15%
Parietal	10% to 12%
Sphenoidal	~2%

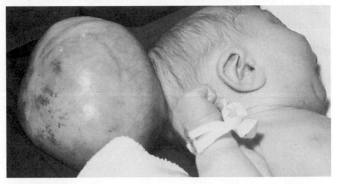

Encephalocele. *(From Zitelli BJ, Davis HW:* Atlas of Pediatric Physical Diagnosis, *ed. 5, Philadelphia, 2007, Mosby.)*

Signs and Symptoms

Frontoethmoidal
- Corpus callosum agenesis
- Hypertelorism
- Interhemispheric lipoma or heterotopias
- Mass almost always contains blood
- Mass near the dorsum of the nose, orbits, or forehead
- Midline craniofacial dysraphism

Parietal
- Aqueduct stenosis
- Arnold-Chiari II malformation (see p. 26)
- Dandy-Walker cysts
- Hydrocephalus
- Microcephaly

Sphenoidal
- Occult and frequently not detected unless computed tomography (CT) and/or magnetic resonance imaging (MRI) of the head is indicated/undertaken

Medical Management

Treatment depends heavily on the size, content, and location of the defect. Surgical correction is the definitive intervention, the ease of which is determined by the size and location of the defect. The best prognosis is found with an anteriorly located encephalocele that is devoid of brain tissue and without any associated anomaly. The poorest prognosis is found in cases with large and/or posterior defects with one or more associated anomalies. Anterior encephaloceles have an almost 100% survival rate, whereas survival rates decline to about 55% in cases of posterior encephaloceles.

Only about 21% of diagnosed cases of encephaloceles are born alive; only about 50% of those neonates live, with only approximately 10% of encephalocele patients surviving the perinatal/neonatal period. Some form of mental deficit is diagnosed in three out of four encephalocele patients who survive birth and surgical correction.

Complications

- Cerebrospinal fluid leak
- Hemorrhage
- Infection
- Meningitis

Anesthesia Implications

Surgical correction of the defect is engaged as soon as feasible after birth. As such, age-appropriate concerns for separation are important, in this case directed more toward the child's parents. The youngest child (days old) will experience less separation anxiety than one who is several months old. The anxiety of the parents will be high no matter the child's age. These parents will benefit most by seeing an anesthetist who is comfortable in dealing with and caring for a very young child. Calm confidence and comfort with caring for this child will be of utmost importance in gaining the trust of this child's parents. The anesthetist should take time to sit with the child's parents and answer any questions and address any concerns the parents may bring up. Talking about their understanding of the proposed surgery will also help alleviate some measure of their anxiety. At the appropriate time, the anesthetist should confidently assume the custody of the child and proceed to the operating room.

Obtaining/maintaining a secure airway, particularly mask fit, may be difficult owing to the size and location of the encephalocele. For example, a true frontal encephalocele may render mask fit almost impossible and inhalation induction may not be possible. The anesthetist may find it necessary to be "creative" with placement of the mask to accomplish the inhalation induction of this infant. Once somnolence is achieved, intravenous access can be obtained and the induction/intubation process completed in a timely fashion.

Occipital encephalocele may cause the child's head to be awkwardly positioned if the child is supine. The anesthetist may find it necessary to turn the child's head to one side or the other so as not to place undue pressure on the defect; it may, in fact, be necessary to place the child's head on a soft foam or gel "doughnut" to remove pressure from the defect. It may also be advisable to attempt intubation with the child in a lateral decubitus position.

Nasal intubation should not be attempted in the child suspected or known to have a sphenoidal encephalocele, which may not be immediately obvious but is normally detected within the first 10 years of life.

Fluid requirements and replacements must be strictly determined and adhered to because of the patient's age.

Blood loss can be relatively large, depending on the size and location of the defect. The age and overall health of the patient, including the presence of any associated systemic anomalies, will have a significant impact on the patient's ability to tolerate blood loss. Large occipital or sphenoidal encephaloceles are of particular importance because they are associated with greater volumes of blood loss. The anesthetist may be called upon to induce deliberate hypotension, with or without hyperventilation, to "relax" the brain and reduce the volume of the encephalocele sac.

A large occipital encephalocele may impede any head/neck extension during the intubation process, making direct laryngoscopy more difficult, and may thus contribute to the inability to intubate the patient with encephalocele. It is prudent to have the pediatric difficult airway cart at hand. In addition, it may be prudent to have a surgeon present to surgically secure the patient's airway if direct laryngoscopy and other measures are unsuccessful.

Epidermolysis Bullosa

Definition

Epidermolysis bullosa (EB) is a group of disorders that give rise to blister formation secondary to even the most minor mechanical trauma.

Incidence

In the United States the incidence of EB is about 50:1,000,000 live births. Internationally it varies according to country, e.g., Norway: 54:1,000,000; Japan: 7.8:1,000,000; Croatia: 9.6:1,000,000.

Etiology

The skin and oral mucosa are composed of several stratified squamous epithelial tissues that contain a basement membrane zone (BMZ). The BMZ itself is composed of specialized components. These components combine to make various complexes that anchor the BMZ. EB results from inherited defects in the BMZ and/or anchoring complexes, depending on the variant of EB.

Signs and Symptoms

- Anal stenosis
- Blisters (conjunctival, oral, genital mucosa)
- Corneal scarring
- Esophageal strictures and webs
- Flexion contractures
- Hyperhidrosis
- Palmoplantar hyperkeratosis
- Phimosis
- Scar-like papules on the trunk
- Urethral stenosis

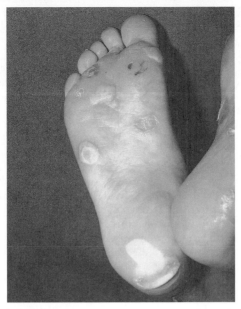

Epidermolysis Bullosa. Epidermolysis bullosa simplex, Weber-Cockayne type. *(From Weston WL, Lane AT, Morelli JB:* Color Textbook of Pediatric Dermatology, *ed. 4, St Louis, 2007, Mosby.)*

Medical Management

The chief concerns with EB are infection and wound healing. Large bullae can form from relatively minor trauma, producing large areas of denuded skin. These areas are generally moist and rich with substrate supportive of bacterial growth. The patient with EB is more susceptible to sepsis as a result.

Strict adherence to hand washing and asepsis are high priorities when dealing with the patient with EB. Any and all wounds must be carefully observed for slow healing or nonhealing.

Dysphagia commonly occurs in the patient with EB and can contribute to formation of esophageal lesions. Oral steroids are combined with phenytoin to reduce the dysphagia and potential for lesion formation.

Good oral hygiene is absolutely essential in the patient with EB. Nevertheless, the patient frequently develops dental caries as the result of enamel defects. Mild saline mouthwashes are recommended rather than those containing alcohol.

Surgical interventions specific to the patient with EB are sometimes required. For example, correction of mitten deformity of the hand(s), esophageal dilation, or squamous cell carcinoma excision may be needed. The patient with EB is susceptible to significant hemodynamic and metabolic alterations. However, intake and absorption may be altered as the result of oral, oropharyngeal, and/or gastrointestinal lesions.

The patient with EB may need physical therapy to combat formation of contractures. Because of the pain and scarring associated with this disease, the patient is more prone to reduced activity levels or frank inactivity, which can further contribute to contracture formation.

Complications

- Chronic blepharitis
- Cicatricial conjunctivitis
- Corneal erosions
- Corneal ulcerations/ scarring
- Dysphagia
- Esophageal webbing/ stricture/stenosis
- Eyelid lesions
- Obliteration of lacrimal ducts
- Pseudosyndactyly
- Squamous cell carcinoma

Anesthesia Implications

The patient with EB is often treated with corticosteroids. Therefore the patient should receive a perioperative dose of hydrocortisone.

The patient who has severe dysphagia may have compromised airway reflexes with the concomitant increased risk of aspiration during either induction and/or emergence.

There have been reports of patients with EB who have significant tracheal stenosis. A thorough noninvasive or minimally invasive airway evaluation should be completed preoperatively, especially if there is any history of airway compromise or demonstrated airway compromise symptoms.

The patient with EB is exquisitely sensitive to skin injury. Any manner of shear force can produce significant injury. Shearing force can be produced by a number of actions during anesthesia. Blood pressure cuff inflation/deflation produces shear forces and should only be placed on the patient after cast padding has been applied. The blood pressure cuff should be monitored to ensure proper function, because a malfunctioning blood pressure cuff that produces excessive and/or sustained inflation will also produce injury. Electrocardiography pads are in essence a form of tape and will produce injury. Tape removal in any form will produce shearing forces and cause injury where it is applied. Commercially available products for securing the endotracheal tube without tape should therefore be used for the patient with EB. Transferring the patient from the OR bed to the stretcher or hospital bed must be accomplished with utmost care and gentleness. Whenever the patient can accomplish transfers, that is preferred in order to minimize, if not avoid, shearing forces.

General and regional anesthesia have been utilized with patients with EB. Regional anesthesia is an appropriate choice for obstetric patients if the skin at the injection site is normal.

Airway management is a cause for concern. Providing general anesthesia via the external mask for a prolonged time period can produce significant facial injury that can be disfiguring. Placement of a laryngeal mask airway (LMA) can produce significant injury to the oral and oropharyngeal tissues and is probably best avoided. Direct laryngoscopy for endotracheal intubation may also produce significant injury to the airway structures: the epiglottis, base of the tongue, glottic folds, and posterior oropharynx. The smallest size endotracheal tube possible should be used for the patient with EB and copious amounts of water-soluble lubricant should be applied to the tube to reduce the possibility of injury to the vocal cords.

Fluid resuscitation and medication injection must be done with care. Overly aggressive fluid delivery or medication injection pressure can be the cause of infiltration of the IV line, which in turn may cause skin lesions. The patency of the intravenous line must be verified on a continual basis. Extravasation of fluids and/or medications in the patient with EB can cause serious injury.

E

Fabry's Disease

Definition

Fabry's disease is a genetic, congenital, X-linked disorder of glycosphingolipid metabolism that is progressive, destructive, and potentially fatal.

Incidence

Internationally, among males, the incidence of Fabry's disease is 1:40,000 to 1:60,000. Among all live births it is 1:80,000 to 1:117,000. Because Fabry's disease is an X-linked inherited disease, it is males who are affected almost exclusively.

Etiology

Alpha-galactosidase A (α-GAL A) deficiency results from an abnormality on the long arm of the X chromosome, specifically Xq22.

Signs and Symptoms

- Acroparesthesias (episodic and chronic)
- Angiokeratomas
- Aplasia
- Cardiomegaly
- Conduction defects
- Diplopia
- Dysarthria
- Hemianopia
- Hemiparesis
- Internuclear ophthalmoplegia
- Left ventricular hypertrophy
- Lens opacities
- Myocardial infarction
- Nystagmus
- Peripheral neuropathy
- Progressive renal failure
- Proteinuria
- Retinal and conjunctival vascular malformations
- Sensory loss
- Valvular deficiencies
- Vertigo

Medical Management

The chronic joint pain associated with Fabry's disease is frequently treated with corticosteroid medications. If the steroid therapy is inadequate or ineffective, alternative pharmacologic therapy may consist of phenytoin, diphenylhydantoin, carbamazepine, or gabapentin.

Replacement of the deficient enzyme, alpha-galactosidase, is highly touted and reportedly works well.

Gastrointestinal aspects of Fabry's disease have been shown to improve with the administration of the prokinetic drug metoclopramide.

Antiplatelet medications have been administered to prevent secondary stroke, but efficacy has not been demonstrated. Embolic concerns originating from cardiac manifestations of Fabry's disease may be treated with anticoagulants.

The patient with Fabry's disease may be treated for renal failure associated with the disease. Kidney transplantation is indicated for renal failure; however, the progressive nature of the disease may continue unabated through other organ systems.

Transplantation of fetal liver is an experimental procedure that has been tried in a small number of patients. This surgical intervention is undertaken with extreme caution.

Complications

- Dementia
- Hypertrophic cardiomyopathy
- Intracranial hemorrhage
- Left ventricular hypertrophy
- Pulmonary hypertension
- Renal failure
- Seizures

Anesthesia Implications

The patient should undergo a comprehensive preoperative eye examination to determine the degree of ophthalmic changes that have occurred as a result of the disease. This will facilitate identification of any ocular changes that result from surgical positioning and/or intraoperative hemodynamic extremes. The patient with Fabry's disease frequently develops lens opacity because of the disease.

The patient's blood urea nitrogen and creatinine levels should be measured preoperatively to determine the degree of renal dysfunction that has been caused by the disease.

A preoperative electroradiogram and echocardiogram should be performed to determine the presence of any myocardial ischemia, valvular lesions, congestive heart failure, or ventricular outflow tract obstruction. A pharmacologic cardiac stress test may be needed for a patient in whom significant coronary disease is suspected, particularly with a sedentary patient. Cardiac catheterization may be necessary if pulmonary hypertension is indicated by an abnormal echocardiogram or if the stress test results are abnormal.

The patient's temperature regulation may be abnormal as a result of lipid accumulation in the brainstem and cerebellar tissues. Methods to actively warm and/or cool the patient should be readily available.

The anesthetist should have drugs prepared in advance and immediately at hand to treat both sudden hypotension as well as sudden hypertension. In a patient with Fabry's disease autonomic neuropathy is highly probable.

Oropharyngeal lesions may be present and may interfere with securing the airway. The selection of the agent for maintenance of general anesthesia should be determined by the patient's co-morbidity(ies).

Postoperative pain control may be difficult and may depend on the effectiveness of medications administered preoperatively. If morphine effectively controlled pain preoperatively, it may be successful postoperatively. If the patient requires the addition of carbamazine or phenytoin for successful pain control, that regimen should continue postoperatively.

A patient who takes carbamazepine or phenytoin regularly may metabolize nondepolarizing muscle relaxants more quickly than other patients. Dosing and re-dosing should be guided by the use of a peripheral nerve stimulator.

Regional anesthesia is a useful and viable alternative for a patient with Fabry's disease. The anesthetist must realize that hemodynamic instability associated with the sympathectomy produced by the blockade may be exaggerated by the patient's autoimmune instability. However, for a patient with progressive lesions of the central nervous system, central blocking techniques are relatively contraindicated.

Patient temperature should be monitored closely. The patient should not be subjected to environmental temperature extremes. The ambient temperature should be stable because of the potential precipitation of acute febrile episodes and/or extremity pain, especially in a patient who exhibits hypohidrosis.

Anticholinergic medications should be avoided in a patient who exhibits hypohidrosis.

F

Facioscapulohumeral Dystrophy

Definition

Facioscapulohumeral dystrophy (FSHD) is a relatively benign, autosomal dominant form of muscular dystrophy that produces marked atrophy of the facial musculature, shoulder girdle, and arm. Facioscapulohumeral dystrophy is also known as Landouzy-Dejerine dystrophy.

Incidence

The incidence of FSHD is approximately 1:20,000. It is the third-most common muscular dystrophy, with a higher frequency in males than females.

Etiology

The specific genetic defect that produces FSHD is not yet known. Several mechanisms have been proposed, including:
1. Position variegation effect on a proximal gene(s)
2. Mutation of a functional gene within the Kpnl repeat units
3. A mitochondrial dysfunction
4. Increased susceptibility to myoblastic oxidative stress

Signs and Symptoms

- Anterior axillary fold upward slope
- Asymmetrical weakness
- Difficulty drinking through a straw
- Difficulty with labial sounds and whistling
- Facial muscle weakness
- Footdrop gait
- Weak scapular fixation
- Weakness of anterior tibialis muscle

F

Facioscapulohumeral Dystrophy. At rest **(A)** and with the arms exerting forward pressure **(B)**. *(From Perkin GD:* Mosby's Color Atlas and Text of Neurology, *ed. 2, Edinburgh, 2002, Mosby.)*

Medical Management

There is no definitive therapy for treatment of FSHD. There have been a few reports of use of albuterol; in one report an oral sustained-release form of the drug was given for 3 months and produced a 12% increase in muscle strength. Another study was a double-blind, placebo-controlled randomized trial of two strengths of albuterol, which demonstrated no improvement in global strength but reported that muscle mass and grip strength improved.

Complications

- Atrial arrest
- Bundle branch block
- Coats' disease
- Dilated cardiomyopathy
- Epilepsy
- Hearing loss (possibly unilateral)
- Labile hypertension
- Mental impairment

Anesthesia Implications

The most relevant physiologic concern for the anesthetist is the patient's diminution of vital capacity. This reduction is related to the weakness of respiratory accessory muscles. The patient with FSHD is likely to have recurrent upper-respiratory infections. The anesthetist should carefully auscultate the chest and inquire about any upper-respiratory symptoms or infections the patient may have. As with any other elective procedure, the surgery is best postponed until appropriate treatment can be completed and the infection can be resolved. As a result of the reduced vital capacity because of the weakness of the accessory muscles, development of atelectasis is a concern. To avert the development of atelectasis, a small amount of positive end-expiratory pressure (PEEP), such as 3 to 5 cm H_2O, may be effective.

Fanconi Syndrome

Definition

Fanconi syndrome is an autosomal recessive, inherited disorder characterized by pancytopenia, bone marrow hypoplasia, and patchy brown skin discolorations resulting from melanin deposits. The melanin deposits are associated with multiple anomalies of the musculoskeletal and genitourinary systems.

Incidence

A true estimate of the frequency of Fanconi syndrome is not available. This disorder develops in association with several conditions, either inherited or acquired.

Etiology

Fanconi syndrome can be inherited, secondary, or idiopathic. The idiopathic form does not have an identifiable cause. Some cases are inherited.

Causes of Fanconi Syndrome	
• Cystinosis	• Heavy metal exposure (cadmium, lead, mercury, platinum, uranium)
• Drug ingestion (tetracycline toxicity, aminoglycosides, cisplatin, ifosfamide, 6-mercaptopurine, valproic acid)	• Hereditary fructose intolerance
	• Inborn error of amino acid and carbohydrate metabolism
• Dysproteinemias	• Lowe syndrome
• Galactosemia	• Mitochondrial cytopathies
• Glycogen storage disorders (e.g., Fanconi-Bickel syndrome*)	• Type I tyrosinemia
	• Wilson's disease (see p. 355)

*See Appendix G: Rare Syndromes.

Signs and Symptoms

- Acidosis
- Dehydration
- Growth failure
- Hypokalemia
- Hypophosphatemia
- Osteomalacia (adults)
- Polydipsia
- Polyuria
- Proteinuria
- Rickets (children)

Medical Management

Management of Fanconi syndrome is predicated on the manifested symptoms. Dehydration resulting from polyuria should be prevented. Free access to water is essential. Treatment should be provided via oral and/or parenteral fluid administration.

Metabolic acidosis is generally corrected with 3 to 10 mg/kg/day of sodium bicarbonate in divided doses. A diuretic may be administered to avoid volume overload, but this causes increased potassium wasting, which must be treated with potassium supplements.

Metabolic acidosis treatment/correction is helpful but is not sufficient for the treatment of bone involvement. The bone involvement must be treated with phosphate and vitamin D supplements.

Liver or kidney transplantation may be necessary to treat the failure of either organ.

Complications

- Congenital cataracts
- Glaucoma
- Hypothyroidism
- Liver failure
- Mental retardation
- Psychiatric disorders
- Renal failure
- Visual impairment

Anesthesia Implications

Fanconi syndrome can result from heavy metal poisoning. Heavy metals can interfere with the metabolism of nondepolarizing muscle relaxants.

Dehydration is a real risk at any time in the patient with Fanconi syndrome. As a result, NPO duration should be kept to the safest tolerable minimum time.

The patient treated with diuretic therapy should also have the electrolyte levels determined immediately before surgery, paying particular attention to the potassium concentration. Potassium supplementation may be required.

Arterial blood gas analysis may be needed in conjunction with monitoring the electrolyte levels to determine the current state of acid-base balance. The patient with Fanconi syndrome is susceptible to bicarbonate loss resulting in metabolic acidosis. The patient's system may attempt to compensate by inducing respiratory alkalosis. This situation needs to be monitored to ensure that the altered respiratory pattern during general anesthesia does not exacerbate the metabolic acidosis. Adequate ventilation during general anesthesia may require supplemental administration of sodium bicarbonate and should be guided by serial arterial blood gas analyses during anesthesia.

Because of the potential need for multiple blood samples, insertion of an arterial pressure line may be appropriate (even considerate) for the patient.

Liver function testing is of particular concern for the patient with long-term Fanconi syndrome, especially those with associated Wilson's disease (p. 355) or tyrosinemia.

The patient may be developmentally delayed and have significant speech impairment due to associated galactosemia. Therefore extra effort and patience may be required of the anesthetist to foster patient understanding and cooperation before administering the anesthetic.

Because of the patient's possibly altered NPO status as well as the potential for renal failure, general anesthesia should be accomplished via rapid sequence induction.

Selection of the volatile agent for maintenance of general anesthesia should be guided by the patient's degree of renal involvement or dysfunction. Regional anesthesia may be appropriate, but fluid resuscitation must be tempered by the degree of renal dysfunction.

Metabolism of various anesthesia-related medications, from nondepolarizing muscle relaxants to midazolam to opioid analgesics, may be altered as a result of the degree of liver dysfunction.

Felty Syndrome

Definition

Felty syndrome is a potentially serious condition associated with seropositive rheumatoid arthritis. It is characterized by rheumatoid arthritis along with splenomegaly and granulocytopenia.

Incidence

Felty syndrome is closely associated with rheumatoid arthritis, which affects about 1% of the general population. Of this 1%, Felty syndrome develops in about 1% to 3%. Therefore the estimated frequency is about 0.01% to 0.03% of the general population. Women are affected at a 3:1 ratio compared to men. It affects Caucasians more than any other race.

Etiology

The pathophysiologic origin of Felty syndrome is not fully understood. Granulocytes coated with immune complexes, diminished granulocyte growth factor levels, and circulating autoantibodies have been demonstrated, as well as linkages to a human leukocyte antigen genotype, suggesting a genetic contribution to development of the disorder.

Signs and Symptoms

- Episcleritis
- Extremity ischemia
- Hepatomegaly
- Joint deformities
- Lower extremity ulcers
- Lymphadenopathy
- Mononeuritis multiplex
- Peripheral neuropathy
- Periungual infarcts
- Pleuritis
- Portal hypertension
- Rheumatoid nodules
- Sjögren syndrome (see p. 316)
- Splenomegaly
- Synovitis
- Weight loss

Medical Management

Treatment of Felty syndrome relies heavily on treatment of the underlying rheumatoid arthritis. Traditionally this regimen has used gold salts as the pharmacologic mainstay. Response to these compounds is slow, however, and methotrexate has supplanted the gold salts in treating both rheumatoid arthritis and Felty syndrome. Cyclophosphamide may be useful in refractory cases, but the potential for leukopenia places distinct limitations on its use.

Etanercept and infliximab are being used to treat rheumatoid arthritis. Both act by blocking the effects of tumor necrosis factor–alpha. Neither has found a definite niche in the treatment of Felty syndrome.

Corticosteroids, specifically methylprednisolone, are frequently used to treat rheumatoid arthritis. The effectiveness is limited by time. The increased potential of infection has demoted these medications to second-line status in the treatment regimen.

Patients with intractable disease, who do not exhibit improvement via these other measures, may be recommended for splenectomy. Despite splenectomy, about 25% of patients experience recurrence of granulocytopenia.

Complications

- Bronchiolitis obliterans
- Congestive heart failure
- Gastrointestinal bleeding
- Immunosuppressive regimen toxicity
- Interstitial pneumonitis
- Life-threatening infection
- Myocarditis
- Pericarditis
- Pneumothorax
- Portal hypertension
- Pulmonary hypertension
- Ruptured spleen

Anesthesia Implications

Because of the close association of Felty syndrome with rheumatoid arthritis, the cervical spine, laryngeal structures, and temporomandibular joints are of particular interest to the anesthetist. Atlantoaxial subluxation is a potential complication during direct laryngoscopy. Symptoms of cervical lesions include occipital headache, nonspecific neck pain and/or stiffness, and stocking-glove distribution paresthesias.

Direct laryngoscopy may prove difficult secondary to severe limitation of the temporomandibular joints' range of motion. Assessment of neck and jaw ranges of motion is essential in the preoperative evaluation of a patient with Felty syndrome.

The patient may have a restrictive lung disease, an obstructive disease, or a combination of both, which will be demonstrated by pulmonary function testing performed preoperatively. Pulmonary effects of rheumatoid arthritis include diffuse interstitial pneumonitis and fibrosis, pleurisy, pleural effusions, necrobiotic nodules, bronchiolitis obliterans, pulmonary arteritis, and apical fibrocavitary lesions. Because of these effects, the patient with Felty syndrome may develop pulmonary hypertension and pneumothorax. These pulmonary effects may also reduce the diffusing capacity of the patient. Restrictive effects can result in the loss of chest wall compliance.

F

Fibrous Dysplasia

Definition

Fibrous dysplasia is a dysplastic bone disorder wherein imma-
ture woven bone forms directly from abnormal fibrous connective tissue. Fibro-osseous tissue within affected bones expands
as a lesion of growing bone. The term "dysplasia" refers to the
person's inability to form mature lamellar bone.

Incidence

The true incidence is not known, but there are estimates that
about 10% of benign bone tumors are the result of fibrous
dysplasia.

Etiology

Fundamentally fibrous dysplasia appears to be a disorder of
postnatal cancellous bone maintenance or an abnormality of
bone-forming mesenchyme.

Signs and Symptoms

- Abnormal cutaneous pig-
  mentation
- Albright syndrome
- Cushing's disease
- Hyperparathyroidism
- Hyperthyroidism
- Hypophosphatemic rickets
- Painful swelling and/or
  deformity of weakened
  bone
- Pathologic fracture(s)
- Precocious puberty

Medical Management

Care and management of a patient with fibrous dysplasia are
generally conservative, with the primary goal to prevent deformity.

Any associated endocrine anomaly should be managed
primarily. These include hyperparathyroidism, hyperthyroidism,
and Cushing's disease.

There is no specific medical treatment for the bone disease.
Some data suggest that administration of vitamin D plus bisphosphonates are at least somewhat effective in pain amelioration and

reconstitution of lesions with normal bone (after physeal closure has occurred). The bony defect may be surgically treated by curettage and allograft or cortical autograft replacement of the lesion. Both allograft and cortical autograft are more resistant to resorption and substitution by dysplastic bone.

Bone deformities, especially of long bones and weight-bearing bones, generally require stabilization. Stabilization is optimally achieved using intramedullary nail fixation. At times, expendable bones with lesions and/or deformities may be treated appropriately by excision.

Complications

- Autonomic hyperreflexia
- Deformity
- Fractures
- Malignant transformation

Anesthesia Implications

Underlying endocrine disorder/dysfunction should be ascertained preoperatively. Appropriate anesthesia concerns will be predicated on the underlying endocrine dysfunction.

Maxillary and/or mandibular involvement may be extensive. Craniofacial deformities may be grotesque. As a result, airway management may be precarious and difficult. Direct laryngoscopy may be difficult to impossible to perform, particularly in a patient with extensive dysplasia of the maxilla and/or mandible. Even fiberoptic laryngoscopy may prove difficult. It is prudent to have a surgeon standing by to surgically secure the airway if necessary.

The patient's bones are extremely fragile—fractures may occur with even the slightest trauma. Correct positioning and adequate padding of the extremities are essential.

Regional anesthesia techniques may be used, but extreme caution must be taken with a patient who has spinal cord lesions.

Autonomic hyperreflexia is possible in a patient with spinal cord lesions, and can give rise to a host of potential anesthesia implications and concerns.

Friedreich's Ataxia

Definition

Friedreich's ataxia is an ataxia inherited via an autosomal recessive gene. This is the most common autosomal recessive form of ataxia, accounting for about half of all hereditary ataxia cases.

Incidence

The incidence of Friedreich's ataxia is estimated at 1:22,000 to 1:50,000, predominately in populations of Europeans and North Americans of European descent. This disorder is virtually nonexistent among African and Asian populations.

Etiology

Friedreich's ataxia is produced by a mutation at the 9q13-21.1 location of chromosome 9, which results in excessive repetitions of the DNA sequence guanine-adenine-adenine (GAA). The onset and length of time until the patient is unable to ambulate is determined by the number of GAA repetitions within the mutation.

Signs and Symptoms

- Absent lower extremity deep tendon reflexes
- Areflexia
- Cardiac enlargement
- Deafness
- Dementia (uncommon)
- Diabetes mellitus
- Difficulty standing and running
- Dysarthria
- Dysphagia
- Facial muscle weakening
- Foot deformity
- Foot inversion
- Hammertoes
- Heart block
- High plantar arches
- Hypertrophic cardiomyopathy
- Incoordination of breathing, speaking, swallowing, and laughing
- Kyphosis
- Mental retardation (uncommon)
- Myocardial fibrosis
- Myocarditis
- Nystagmus
- Pes cavus
- Pes varus

- Progressive cardiac failure
- Progressively slow and clumsy walking
- Psychosis (uncommon)
- Scoliosis
- Swallowing weakness
- Systolic ejection murmurs
- Tachycardia
- Ventricular hypertrophy

Medical Management

The prognosis for the patient with Friedreich's ataxia is not promising. No reported treatment regimens are known to alter the progressively detrimental neurologic nature of this disease. Present treatment regimens are oriented toward associated systemic problems, such as heart failure, cardiac dysrhythmias, or diabetes mellitus.

Surgical interventions are essentially palliative in nature. Surgical correction of scoliosis or deformities of a foot (or feet) may be undertaken in a select few patients to lessen their discomfort and ease respiratory symptoms brought on by the scoliosis. No definitive surgical option produces a cure for Friedreich's ataxia or halts the progression.

The disease generally lasts 15 to 20 years. Patients generally survive to age 25 to 30 years. The typical age of onset is between 8 and 15 years old. Occasionally, a patient with Friedreich's ataxia who does not have heart disease or diabetes mellitus may survive into the sixth or seventh decade of life, but that is the exception rather than the rule.

Complications

- Cardiomyopathy
- Congestive heart failure
- Infections
- Kyphoscoliosis
- Pes cavus
- Pressure sores

Anesthesia Implications

Pulmonary assessment is a crucial preoperative task along with cardiac evaluation. Restrictive pulmonary disease frequently develops in association with Friedreich's ataxia. Cardiomyopathy is also frequently seen in Friedreich's ataxia. The choice of volatile agent for the patient will be heavily influenced by the degree of cardiac and pulmonary dysfunction. It is desirable to use an agent that relaxes the bronchial smooth muscles, such as sevoflurane. Hemodynamic support is highly desired, such as is provided by desflurane. Positive pressure ventilation for the patient with Friedreich's ataxia must take into account the lack of lung compliance resulting from the disease. Reduced inspiratory pressures along with prolonged expiratory phases will reduce the risk of pulmonary injury.

The effects of nondepolarizing muscle relaxants have been reported to be altered by this disease process. The anesthetist must be mindful of the similarities of this disease process to other motor neuron degeneration diseases. Typically both onset and recovery from nondepolarizing muscle relaxants will at first appear to be within the expected limits; however, preoperative preparation should be made for prolonged ventilatory support for the patient because of the probable residual effects of any muscle relaxants following the surgical procedure.

Regional anesthesia techniques have been reported to be effective in patients with Friedreich's ataxia without exacerbating neurologic symptoms.

The anesthetist should anticipate and expect any of a variety of cardiac dysrhythmias as a result of the high degree of associated cardiomyopathies, particularly hypertrophic myopathies.

Galactosemia

Definition

Galactosemia is an inherited metabolic deficiency of the galactose-1-phosphate uridyltransferase enzyme. This is one of the most common carbohydrate metabolism disorders and may be life threatening or even fatal in the neonatal period.

Incidence

The incidence of galactosemia in the United States is about 1:40,000 to 1:60,000 people; worldwide the incidence varies considerably. All races and ethnic groups can be affected, with the Asian population having the lowest occurrence of the disease.

Etiology

Galactosemia results from alteration of the gene for galactose-1-phosphate uridyltransferase (GALT) found at the 9p13 band.

Signs and Symptoms

- Ascites
- Ataxia
- Bleeding coagulopathy
- Cataracts
- Hepatomegaly
- Hypergonadotropic hypo-gonadism
- Hypotonia
- Jaundice
- Lethargy
- Liver dysfunction
- Poor growth
- Sepsis
- Tremor
- Vitreous hemorrhage

Medical Management

The primary treatment is elimination of lactose from the patient's diet. Routine screening of newborns generally initiates the diagnosis of this disease. This is particularly important for the newborn being breastfed, since breast milk is high in lactose. Before lactose is eliminated from the diet, an infant with galactosemia exhibits poor growth over the first weeks of life.

Galactose-1-phosphate accumulates quite rapidly in the affected infant; if untreated, this accumulation can lead to cataracts, cirrhosis, and severe mental retardation.

Complications

- Ascites
- Cataracts
- Cirrhosis
- Cognitive impairment
- Hypergonadotropic hypo-
  gonadism
- Primary ovarian failure
- Speech impairment
- Vitreous hemorrhage

Anesthesia Implications

Anesthesia care is greatly affected by the degree of liver dysfunction in these patients. Numerous anesthesia medications are metabolized to a great degree, if not exclusively, by the liver. The anesthetist must anticipate a prolongation of the effects of such medications, and prudence would thus dictate reducing their dosage(s). The anesthetist should also anticipate the need for postoperative ventilatory support secondary to residual effects of medications.

The newly diagnosed neonate may have prolonged/elevated clotting times. Such a patient may lose an inordinately large amount of blood during a surgical procedure. Circulating volume, fluid resuscitation, and blood loss replacement are critical perioperative evaluations that must be completed.

A patient who is jaundiced should have the hemoglobin concentration determined preoperatively.

The patient may have albuminuria, resulting in an osmotic diuresis. As a result, the patient's urine output should not be relied on very heavily as an indicator of intravascular volume.

Gardner Syndrome

Definition

Gardner syndrome is a type of familial adenomatous polyposis that also has extracolonic manifestations, including intestinal polyposis, desmoids, osteomas, and epidermoid cysts. The disorder is inherited via an autosomal dominant pattern.

Incidence

The incidence of Gardner syndrome is about 1:7000 live births, of which 80% are of mendelian dominant inheritance and 20% are spontaneous mutations.

Etiology

Gardner syndrome develops as the result of five mutations:
1. Mutation of the APC gene
2. Loss of DNA methylation
3. RAS gene mutation on chromosome 12
4. Deletion of the colon cancer (DCC) gene on chromosome 18
5. TP53 gene mutation on chromosome 17

Signs and Symptoms

- Adrenal carcinoma
- Biliary duct carcinoma
- Congenital hyperpigmentation of the retinal pigment epithelium
- Cushing syndrome
- Desmoid tumor
- Epidermal cysts
- Gastric carcinoma
- Hepatoblastoma
- Impacted teeth
- Multiple colonic polyps
- Multiple duodenal polyps
- Multiple gastric polyps
- Osteoma
- Osteosarcoma
- Periampullary carcinoma
- Root abnormalities
- Sebaceous cysts
- Skin fibromas
- Supernumerary teeth
- Thyroid carcinoma

G

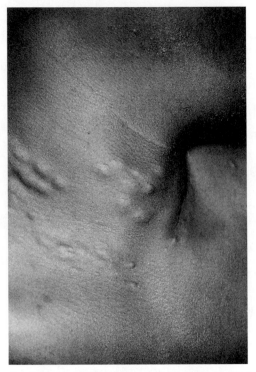

Gardner Syndrome. Multiple epidermoid cysts are present in this patient
with adenomatous colonic polyps. *(From Callen JP, et al:* Dermatological Signs
of Internal Disease, *ed. 3, Philadelphia, 2003, Saunders.)*

Medical Management

The most direct and appropriate treatment for Gardner syndrome is surgical colectomy because 65% of patients have carcinoma at the time of diagnosis.

Surgical Procedures for Gardner Syndrome
• Proctocolectomy with ileostomy • Total colectomy with ileorectal anastomosis • Proctocolectomy with ileal pouch anal anastomosis

Treatment Goals for Gardner Syndrome
• Treat or eliminate colorectal cancer risk • Preserve/maintain continence and defecation abilities • Preserve sexual organ innervation • Reduce mortality and morbidity

Sulindac appears to produce rectal polyp regression for patients who have had total colectomy. Doxorubicin with dacarbazine also reduces polyps following colectomy.

Desmoid polyps of the abdominal wall or extra abdominal manifestations of Gardner syndrome are best treated with sulindac, tamoxifen, or a combination of the two medications.

Complications

- Bowel obstruction
- CHRPE (congenital hypertrophy of retinal pigmented epithelium)
- Colon perforation
- Dental abnormalities
- Desmoid tumor
- Duodenal polyps
- Epidermoid cysts
- Gastric polyps
- Hemorrhage
- Hepatoblastoma
- Osteoma
- Thyroid cancer

Anesthesia Implications

A patient with Gardner syndrome may present with low hemoglobin concentrations and may also lose greater amounts of blood than typical for a given operation. The patient is more apt to require blood transfusion(s).

Dental abnormalities may produce jaw pain. Osteomas may develop in the mandible. Direct laryngoscopy must be undertaken with caution as well as gentleness to minimize airway trauma.

As with any extensive bowel/lower abdominal surgical procedure, fluid resuscitation is a critical issue. Preoperative bowel cleaning preparation combined with fluid intake restrictions can produce significant dehydration. The patient may then be falsely hemoconcentrated.

Thyroid cancer may cause significant alteration to the patient's airway anatomy.

Hepatoblastoma, if present, may alter the metabolism of many anesthesia-related medications, from opioid analgesics to nondepolarizing muscle relaxants. Residual effects of any of these medications, singularly or in combination, may result in the need for postoperative ventilatory support.

Gaucher's Disease

Definition

Gaucher's disease is an autosomal recessive inherited disorder resulting from deficiency of acid beta-glucosidase. It is characterized by thrombocytopenia, anemia, hepatosplenomegaly, and bone pain.

Incidence

The incidence of Gaucher's disease in non-Jewish populations is 1:40,000. For the Ashkenazi Jewish population, the carrier rate is 1:15, whereas the disease rate is 1:855. In those of Norrbottnian Swedish descent, the incidence of Type III Gaucher's disease is 1:50,000.

Etiology

All three types of Gaucher's disease are caused by deficiency of the acid β-glucoside as the result of a mutation in the structural gene providing the enzyme encoding.

Subtypes of Gaucher's Disease
• Type I: Adult/non-neuronopathic form
• Type II: Infantile/acute neuronopathic form
• Type III: Juvenile/Norrbottnian form

Signs and Symptoms

- Ataxia
- Dementia
- Fatigue
- Generalized weakness
- Hepatosplenomegaly
- Pathologic fractures
- Psychomotor retardation
- Seizures
- Severe bone and joint pain
- Spasticity
- Strabismus
- Trismus

Medical Management

The primary focus of medical care for the patient with Gaucher's disease is administration of the enzyme therapy agent imiglucerase. Both visceral and hematologic manifestations of Gaucher's disease respond relatively quickly to enzyme replacement therapy; however, skeletal manifestations of the disease are slow to respond to enzyme therapy. Enzyme replacement therapy is usually directed by a metabolic disease specialist frequently working closely with a hematologist.

Splenomegaly may be treated surgically by splenectomy. This surgical intervention is used less frequently since the development of enzyme replacement therapy.

Not all patients respond favorably to enzyme replacement therapy, particularly those with portal hypertension, extensive splenic infarction, extensive splenic fibrosis, pulmonary manifestations, hematologic malignancy, and/or cirrhosis.

Hip arthroplasty, total or hemi, may be needed secondary to skeletal manifestations of this disease. Prudence dictates re-evaluation of the need for such surgery after several months of enzyme replacement therapy.

Patients with documented splenomegaly are advised to avoid contact sports and other activities/avocations with greatly elevated risk of splenic rupture.

Complications

- Anemia
- Avascular necrosis
- Bony infarcts
- Cirrhosis (rare)
- Esophageal varices
- Fibrotic parenchymal infiltrates
- Hepatomegaly
- Hypergammaglobulinemia
- Impaired neutrophil chemotaxis
- Intrapulmonary vascular dilation
- Leukopenia
- Portal hypertension
- Pulmonary infiltrates
- Splenic rupture
- Thrombocytopenia
- T-lymphocyte deficiency

Anesthesia Implications

Glycosphingolipid deposits in the head and neck may encroach on the oropharynx and trachea and may contribute to a smaller-than-normal mouth, rendering direct laryngoscopy and airway management difficult. These deposits may cause the glottis and/or trachea to be smaller than expected, requiring the anesthetist to reconsider the size of the endotracheal tube and place a smaller one. Placement of a laryngeal mask airway (LMA) may be impeded because of the patient's small mouth opening.

A patient with the infantile/Type II variant of Gaucher's disease may be severely developmentally delayed and also prone to stridor. Hepatosplenomegaly can be very significant in the young patient. The prognosis for the patient with infantile/Type II Gaucher's disease is very poor, with rapid progression culminating in death, usually within 2 years.

Gastroesophageal reflux, aspiration, and the continuing potential for aspiration are closely associated with both Type II and Type III Gaucher's disease; therefore rapid sequence induction is in order for the provision of general anesthesia.

As with any anticipated difficult airway scenario, the difficult airway cart should be readily available and the anesthetist with the most experience should be chosen to attempt intubation. Anesthestists should be prepared to provide postoperative ventilatory support to allow the patient the best opportunity to fully regain control of protective airway reflexes and to recover full muscle tone.

Regional anesthesia is an option for the patient and has been used successfully in the past.

Goodpasture Syndrome

Definition

Goodpasture syndrome is an autoimmune process composed of acute glomerulonephritis in conjunction with pulmonary alveolar hemorrhage and antiglomerular basement membrane antibodies.

Incidence

The incidence of Goodpasture syndrome is approximately 1:100,000. The disease is reported in all races, but occurs most frequently among Caucasians. Males are affected more than females at a ratio of 2.9:1.

Etiology

The cause of Goodpasture syndrome is the production of antiglomerular basement membrane antibodies, frequently as the result of exposure to an environmental insult in genetically predisposed people. The environmental triggers include cigarette smoke, hydrocarbon inhalation, and viral infections.

Signs and Symptoms

- Azotemia
- Bronchial breathing
- Cough
- Cyanosis
- Dyspnea (exertional)
- Edema
- Fatigue/weakness
- Fevers/chills/diaphoresis
- Gross hematuria
- Hemoptysis
- Inspiratory crackles
- Proteinuria
- Tachypnea

Medical Management

Treatment of Goodpasture syndrome involves two simultaneous interventions: (1) removing existing pathogenic antibodies and (2) preventing subsequent production of new antibodies. Antibody removal is best achieved via plasma exchange.

Current recommendations for an adult patient present two options: either daily exchanges for 14 consecutive days or every third day for 1 month. A plasma exchange session involves total volumes of 3 L to 4 L, with volume replacement consisting of albumin and fresh frozen plasma.

Preventing new antibody production is best accomplished via immunosuppression. Immunosuppression therapy usually consists of administering corticosteroids and cyclophosphamide. An adult with serum creatinine levels of 8 generally has a poor renal outcome.

Immunosuppression treatment for a pediatric patient generally consists of 6 months of corticosteroid therapy combined with giving cyclophosphamide for 3 months.

Therapeutic response is monitored by serial measurements of antiglomerular basement membrane antibody titers, serum creatinine levels, and chest x-rays to measure progress and determine the duration of therapeutic interventions.

Sodium restriction may be implemented, particularly for a patient being treated with corticosteroids or a patient with severe proteinuria and nephrotic syndrome. Fluid intake may be restricted, depending on whether the patient's renal function indicates it and whether cyclophosphamide is a component of the treatment regimen.

Liberal fluid intake is encouraged for the patient being treated with cyclophosphamide who has good urine output and stable blood pressure. The goal is to promote continued good urine output and reduce the risk of hemorrhagic cystitis.

Complications

- Anaphylactoid reactions
- End-stage renal disease
- Hemorrhage
- Metabolic alkalosis
- Opportunistic infection (bacterial or fungal)
- Post-transfusion hepatitis
- Recurrent pulmonary hemorrhage
- Thrombosis

Anesthesia Implications

If at all possible, any surgical procedure should be delayed or postponed until the patient's condition is optimized. This is particularly important for a patient whose diagnosis of Goodpasture syndrome is relatively recent or a patient with a long-standing diagnosis but experiencing an acute exacerbation of symptoms. Medical treatment should be well established and any pulmonary problems treated and almost totally resolved before undertaking anything other than fully emergent surgery.

Preoperative evaluation must focus on the function of the pulmonary and renal systems. Blood urea nitrogen, serum creatinine, and urinary output/urinalysis are good indicators of renal function. Pulmonary evaluation should include arterial blood gas analysis, chest x-ray, diffusing capacity, and spirometry. Chest x-rays may demonstrate pulmonary infiltrates bilaterally secondary to alveolar hemorrhage. Hypoxemia and restrictive defects may be demonstrated in patients with ongoing pulmonary involvement.

Preoperative complete blood count may demonstrate microcytic anemia from hemorrhages. The patient may require preoperative blood transfusion, particularly before a large abdominal procedure or one anticipated to involve large volumes of blood loss intraoperatively. The patient is also more apt to require postoperative blood transfusion.

The anemia secondary to hemorrhage has a significant impact on oxygenation. With a low hemoglobin concentration, the O_2-dissociation curve is shifted to the right. If there is an ongoing alveolar hemorrhage, gas exchange is impaired and the anemia will be exacerbated. Any alveolar hemorrhage present can be worsened by use of high fractions of inspired oxygen (Fio_2) and high inspiratory pressures. As a result, oxygen delivery may be further compromised.

Fluid resuscitation should not be overly aggressive to help reduce further antiglomerular basement membrane antibody–mediated damage to the lungs.

Blood pressure should be monitored with an intra-arterial pressure catheter placement, particularly for a patient with anything more than the mildest expression of this disease and/or for a patient scheduled for large, intricate surgical procedures in which large fluid shifts are anticipated.

A pulmonary artery catheter and transesophageal echocardiogram are prudent monitors to include in the care of the patient scheduled for large, intricate surgical procedures and/or one with significant pulmonary manifestations of the disease. Both devices, together or singularly, provide indispensable information to guide the anesthetist in fluid resuscitation and management, both intra- and postoperatively.

The patient's renal status has significant bearing on the selection of the volatile inhalational agent and any intravenous agent. Any medications that are potentially nephrotoxic should be avoided. Medications that depend on renal excretion will necessarily need the dose(s) customized based on the patient's creatinine clearance level.

G

Guillain-Barré Syndrome

Definition

Guillain-Barré syndrome is an acute, ascending motor neuron paralysis that progresses very rapidly. This disease is also called acute inflammatory demyelinating polyradiculoneuropathy (AIDP), acute idiopathic polyneuritis, or acute inflammatory polyneuropathy.

Incidence

The incidence of Guillain-Barré syndrome ranges from 0.5:100,000 to 1.5:100,000. It is reported in all races. This disease has a slightly higher occurrence in males than in females (1.2:1). Risk of the disease increases steadily after age 40 years and peaks at 70 to 80 years.

Etiology

Guillain-Barré syndrome is an autoimmune-mediated malady frequently triggered by environmental factors, which can be pathogenic or stressful exposures. Pathogenic triggers usually precede the onset of symptoms by 1 to 3 weeks. The triggers include Epstein-Barr virus, cytomegalovirus, hepatitis, varicella, *Mycoplasma pneumoniae,* and *Campylobacter jejuni.* Endogenous antigens include myelin P-2, ganglioside GQ1b, GM1, and GT1a.

Signs and Symptoms

- Ataxia
- Autonomic instability
- Dysesthesias
- Illness or immunization 2 to 4 weeks before onset of symptoms
- Ophthalmoplegia
- Orthostatic hypotension
- Pain
- Polyneuritis cranialis
- Progressive ascending flaccid paralysis
- Respiratory compromise
- Urinary retention

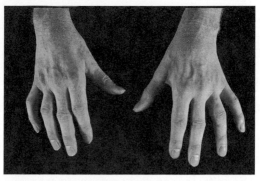

Guillain-Barré Syndrome. Residual hand muscle wasting in Guillain-Barré syndrome. *(From Perkin GD:* Mosby's Color Atlas and Text of Neurology, *ed. 2, Edinburgh, 2002, Mosby.)*

G

Medical Management

Treatment of Guillain-Barré syndrome is primarily focused on immunomodulation and supportive measures. Intravenous immunoglobulin is considered the most effective immuno-modulation therapeutic measure.

Plasmapheresis is also an effective immunomodulation treatment that can significantly shorten the recovery time, but the efficacy is most optimal if initiated within 2 weeks of the appearance of symptoms.

Respiratory muscles are frequently affected by this disease. The patient's ability to maintain adequate respiratory effort is quickly impaired. Mechanical ventilation is indicated when arterial Pco_2 is greater than 50 mm Hg, alveoarterial O_2 tension gradient is greater than 300 mm Hg at an Fio_2 of 1.0, maximum inspiratory and expiratory pressures are less than 30 cm H_2O, and vital capacity is under 14 mL/kg

Autonomic dysfunction also frequently occurs with Guillain-Barré syndrome and is characterized by labile blood pressure—vacillation between hypertension and hypotension—sinus tachycardia, diaphoresis, and orthostatic hypotension. Treatment of the hypertension and hypotension may be required.

Complications

- Adult respiratory distress syndrome
- Autonomic instability
- Constipation
- Decubitus ulcers/pressure sores
- Dysesthesias

- Gastritis
- Ileus
- Pneumonia
- Pulmonary embolus
- Respiratory muscle weakness
- Septicemia

Anesthesia Implications

Chief concerns for the anesthetist revolve around the severity of both respiratory and autonomic dysfunction. Anesthetic management for the patient with Guillain-Barré syndrome incorporates the same concerns as for other patients with degenerative motor neuron disorders. Succinylcholine should not be used in the patient with Guillain-Barré syndrome because of the potassium release associated with its administration. The patient may likely exhibit greater sensitivity to nondepolarizing muscle relaxants.

Because of the associated autonomic dysfunction, intraoperative intra-arterial pressure should be monitored continuously. The catheter should be inserted preoperatively because of the large, rapid fluctuations that may occur, particularly during induction.

No particular inhalational anesthetic agent is more or less desirable or effective than another for the patient with Guillain-Barré syndrome. The anesthetist should anticipate potentially prolonged or residual effects from inhalational agents. The possible residual effects may combine with residual effects of nondepolarizing muscle relaxants to necessitate postoperative ventilation.

Use of regional anesthesia is controversial. A few reports have demonstrated no complications or detrimental effects from this anesthesia technique; however, some reports have suggested that a regional anesthetic can cause onset of this disease.

Homocystinuria

Definition

Homocystinuria is an autosomal recessive disorder of methionine metabolism that produces an abnormal accumulation of homocystine, homocysteine-cysteine complex, and other metabolites in the blood and urine.

Incidence

The incidence of homocystinuria is variable, with reports between 1:50,000 to 1:200,000.

Etiology

Homocystinuria is an autosomal recessive inherited defect in either the transsulfuration pathway or methylation pathway, producing deficiencies of cystathionine beta-synthase enzyme, defective methylcobalamin synthesis, or an abnormality of methylene tetrahydrofolate reductase.

Signs and Symptoms

- Ectopia lentis
- Genu valgum
- Kyphoscoliosis
- Kyphosis
- Marfanoid habitus
- Mental retardation
- Osteoporosis
- Pes carinatum
- Pes excavatum
- Seizures
- Signs and symptoms of stroke (hemiplegia, aphasia, ataxia, pseudobulbar palsy)

Medical Management

The medication of choice for treatment of homocystinuria is pyridoxine, between 100 to 500 mg/day in divided doses. Vitamin B_{12} and folic acid may be added to the treatment regimen if pyridoxine is not effective in controlling the levels of homocystine.

Some patients are sensitive to pyridoxine. In such cases, dietary restrictions on methionine intake are instituted along with administration of betaine supplements to reduce homocystine levels.

Complications

- Deep vein thrombosis
- Hypoglycemia
- Stroke
- Thromboembolism

Anesthesia Implications

Thromboembolism is a major concern for patients with homocystinuria. Vascular occlusion of any major organ (heart, lungs, brain, or kidney) may have devastating consequences.

Hypotension, or low-flow states, must be avoided at all costs. A prophylactic intervention is maintenance of adequate hydration. Accurate determination of fluid requirements is important, but adherence to that administration schedule is essential.

Bleeding times and platelet function must be determined preoperatively. The elevated adhesiveness of the patient's platelets, which increases the risk of thrombus formation, warrants the administration of low-dose aspirin or dipyridamole as a counteraction. Antiembolic stockings and/or sequential pneumatic compression devices should be used as prophylaxis against venous stasis and potential deep vein thrombosis.

The patient with homocystinuria is susceptible to hypoglycemia secondary to hyperinsulinemia, which is triggered by hypermethionemia. Capillary blood glucose should be monitored, typically on an hourly basis, throughout the perioperative period. It may be prudent to include glucose-containing solutions in the fluid replacement regimen.

The patient with osteoporosis requires extra care when being positioned to avoid undue trauma or injury. If possible or feasible, allow the patient to position himself or herself for comfort and safety.

For general anesthesia, the maintenance agent selected should promote high peripheral flow, reduce vascular resistance, maintain cardiac output, and allow for rapid recovery. Regional anesthesia may be employed, but particular attention should be paid to preparatory fluid loading to avoid hypotension resulting from the induced sympathectomy of the regional anesthetic. Instillation of the regional anesthetic may be challenging, particularly in the patient with kyphoscoliosis.

The patient with both kyphoscoliosis and pectus excavatum may demonstrate a pattern of restrictive lung disease. Direct laryngoscopy may be difficult because of the skeletal defects similar to those of Marfan syndrome (p. 216) that may be produced by homocystinuria.

H

Huntington's Chorea

Definition

Huntington's chorea is an incurable, autosomal dominant inherited disorder, with onset as an adult, associated with loss in specific subsets of neurons in the basal ganglia and cortex. This disorder is characterized by involuntary movements, dementia, and behavioral changes.

Incidence

The frequency of Huntington's chorea varies significantly, depending on the particular country or region.

Frequency of Huntington's Chorea by Country/Region	
Country/Region	Incidence
United States	4.1-8.4:100,000
Lake Maracaibo, Venezuela	700:100,000
Mauritius (off South Africa)	46:100,000
Tasmania	17.4:100,000
Europe (most)	1.63-9.95:100,000
Finland	<1:100,000
Japan	<1:100,000

Etiology

The gene for Huntington's chorea, designated IT15, is found on chromosome 4p. Selective neuronal dysfunction and loss of neurons may be explained by several mechanisms, such as excitotoxicity, oxidative stress, impaired energy metabolism, and apoptosis. One theory is that polyglutamine repeats cause neuronal degeneration through interactions with other proteins containing short polyglutamine tracts.

The duration of this disorder is quite variable, but the mean duration is about 19 years. Survival is generally 10 to 25 years after the onset of the illness.

This disorder afflicts both genders without preference. In general, onset occurs between the ages of 35 to 44 years, with a range from 2 years of age to more than 80 years. Onset of this disorder earlier than 10 years of age or later than 70 years is not unheard of, but is rare.

Signs and Symptoms

- Akinetic-rigid syndrome
- Argumentative
- Attention deficit
- Bradykinesia
- Clonus
- Dancing gait
- Dementia
- Depression
- Diminished verbal fluency
- Dramatic weight loss
- Dysarthria
- Dystonia
- Early mental status changes (increased irritability, moodiness, antisocial behavior)
- Erratic behavior
- Facial grimaces
- Fidgetiness
- Impulsive behavior
- Memory disturbances
- Obsessive-compulsive disorder
- Personality changes
- Piano-playing finger motions
- Postural instability
- Psychosis
- Rigidity rather than chorea (in children)
- Seizures
- Sexual disorders
- Sleep disorders/ disturbances
- Slow cognition
- Spasticity
- Suicidal ideation/ tendencies
- Uncontrollable flailing

Medical Management

Huntington's chorea is not curable. Initial interventions are usually nonpharmacologic, directed at establishing and maintaining a safe patient environment. When the patient's chorea advances to the point of dysfunction, administration of some form of benzodiazepine such as diazepam or clonazepam may be beneficial. Dopamine-depleting agents such as reserpine or some neuroleptic medication may prove beneficial as well.

A patient with Huntington's chorea who has significant bradykinesia and rigidity may improve when treated with levodopa or dopamine agonists.

The depression that may accompany Huntington's chorea must be recognized quickly and treated without delay. A selective serotonin reuptake inhibitor is the drug of choice, although bupropion, venlafaxine, nefazodone, and tricyclic antidepressants may be used effectively in some patients. Some patients with refractory depression may benefit from treatment with electroconvulsive therapy (ECT).

A patient who has hallucinations, delusions, and/or schizophrenia-like symptoms may require treatment with antipsychotic medications such as quetiapine, clozapine, olanzapine, or risperidone.

Antidepressants, selective serotonin reuptake inhibitors, mood stabilizers, and possibly atypical neuroleptic agents may be effective in treating the patient's irritability. Mania, obsessive-compulsive disorder, sexual disorders, myoclonus, tics, dystonia, epilepsy, and anxiety are more infrequent characteristics of Huntington's chorea that may need pharmacologic intervention.

Surgical interventions are experimental and have consisted of ablative procedures and fetal cell transplantation; however, insufficient data exist to support these interventions as anything other than experimental procedures at present.

Complications

- Choking
- Difficulty swallowing
- Increased risk for suicide due to depression
- Personality changes
- Progressive, disabling dementia
- Rigidity

Anesthesia Implications

There have been few reports of anesthesia care for patients with Huntington's chorea. There has been a single reported case of prolonged action/delayed recovery from sodium thiopental in a patient with Huntington's chorea; however, there have been no subsequent reports of similar responses to thiopental. The response to midazolam may also be exaggerated.

Rapid sequence or modified rapid sequence induction is recommended for the patient requiring general anesthesia. Rapid sequence induction is indicated because the patient has a greater risk of pulmonary aspiration secondary to dysphagia. For this reason, the patient with Huntington's chorea should be assessed preoperatively to determine the degree of dysphagia that may be present. Anesthesia has been successfully induced without incident using propofol. It has also been successfully used for maintenance of anesthesia. Patients with Huntington's chorea have a significantly higher incidence of reduced pseudocholinesterase activity. As a result, the anesthetist should anticipate a prolonged effect by succinylcholine as well as any other medications metabolized by pseudocholinesterase.

Butyrophenones and/or phenothiazines have been incorporated successfully into the anesthetic regimen to better control choreiform movements during the perioperative period. If an anticholinergic medication is required, the preferred agent is glycopyrrolate, which does not exacerbate the patient's choreiform movements.

The degree of physiologic dysfunction present in the patient with Huntington's chorea will determine other subsequent anesthesia concerns.

Areas of Marked Neuronal Loss in Huntington's Chorea

- Caudate nucleus
- Cerebellum
- Deep layers of the cerebral cortex
- Globus pallidus
- Neostriatum
- Putamen
- Substantia nigra
- Subthalamic nucleus
- Thalamus

Huntington's Chorea Severity Grading

Grade 0: No detectable histologic neuropathology in the presence of a typical clinical picture and positive Huntington's chorea family history

Grade 1: Neuropathologic changes detected microscopically but without gross atrophy

Grade 2: Striatal atrophy present but caudate nucleus is still convex

Grade 3: More severe striatal atrophy, flat caudate nucleus

Grade 4: Most severe striatal atrophy, caudate nucleus medial surface is concave

Hydatid Disease

Definition

Hydatid disease is a parasitic infestation by a tapeworm of the genus Echinococcus.

Incidence

The incidence of hydatid disease in the United States is <1:1,000,000, except in Alaska, where the incidence is <1:100,000. Internationally, the incidence varies relative to the geographic region; endemic areas include countries bordering the Mediterranean Sea, the Middle East, southern South America, Iceland, Australia, New Zealand, and Africa. In these areas, cystic echinococcosis (CE) occurs at 1:100,000 to 220:100,000; alveolar echinococcosis (AE) occurs at 0.03:100,000 to 1.2:100,000. There is no true racial or gender preference for the affliction.

Etiology

Hydatid disease originates with the ingestion, by an intermediate host, of the eggs of larval cestodes of the phylum Platyhelminthes (tapeworm). The eggs hatch into metacastodes, which infest the liver, lungs, muscles, and other organs.

Medically Important Species of Echinococcus	
Species	Disease
Echinococcus granulosus	Cystic echinococcosis (CE)
Echinococcus multilocularis	Alveolar echinococcosis (AE)
Echinococcus vogelii	Rare infestation(s)

Signs and Symptoms

- Abdominal tenderness
- Ascites (rare)
- Blindness (rare)
- Cerebral herniation
- Coma
- Decreased visual acuity (rare)
- Erythema
- Exophthalmos (rare)
- Fever
- Hepatomegaly
- Hypotension
- Jaundice
- Spider angiomas
- Splenomegaly
- Urticaria

Medical Management

Treatment regimens for hydatid disease differ for cystic echino-coccosis (CE) and alveolar echinococcosis (AE).

Cystic Echinococcosis

Surgical excision is the treatment of choice for CE and the only avenue leading to cure of the infestation. A new treatment, called PAIR, is currently being refined. PAIR is an acronym for **P**uncture, **A**spiration, **I**njection, and **R**easpiration. PAIR technique is guided by either ultrasound or computed tomography. It must be accompanied by chemotherapy in the form of benzimidazole for the 4 days preceding the procedure and for 1 to 3 months postprocedure. This technique can be performed on the liver, kidney, or bones, but not in the lungs or brain. Surgical interventions range from radical surgery—a total pericystectomy or partial resection of the affected organ—to conservative procedures, such as open cystectomy, to simple procedures, such as placing a drainage tube to empty infected and communicating cysts. The possibility of relapse decreases with increasing complexity of the surgical treatment.

Alveolar Echinococcus

Radical complete resection of AE cysts, such as lung wedge resection or lobectomy, is the only possible curative intervention for AE patients. Some infestations dictate that total hepatectomy with transplantation be carried out, but only if no extra hepatic disease is present. Parasite re-emergence may occur in the transplanted organ, and distant metastasis may occur in immunosuppressed patients.

H

Complications

- Alopecia
- Anaphylactic shock
- Anemia
- Atelectasis
- Embryotoxicity
- Hemorrhage
- Hepatotoxicity
- Hypoxemia
- Infection
- Metastasis
- Recurrence of infestation
- Sclerosing cholangitis
- Teratogenicity
- Thrombocytopenia
- Tissue damage (PAIR procedure)

Anesthesia Implications

Respiratory compromise may result from larger alveolar cysts. Spirometric evaluation preoperatively will indicate reduced volumes secondary to space-occupying lesions.

Resection of the alveolar cyst requires isolation of the affected lung. One-lung ventilation is generally well tolerated. Atelectasis may be present, particularly in the right lower lobe, because of encroachment by the enlarged liver. The atelectasis results in hypoxemia, which will worsen after anesthesia induction. Positive end-expiratory pressure (PEEP) may be an effective treatment to prevent extension of the atelectasis. When one-lung ventilation is anticipated, placement of an arterial pressure catheter is a prudent measure to assess patient tolerance of the method via serial arterial blood gas analysis.

Liver dysfunction may interfere with metabolic functions. As a result, actions of medications may be prolonged, depending on how effectively the liver metabolizes medications.

Good, continuous communication between surgeon and anesthetist is essential. Paralysis is essential, especially during drainage and delivery of the cyst(s), to avoid movement and spillage of the cyst contents. If the cyst contents are spilled, anaphylaxis and shock may result. Because of these extreme consequences, preoperative intravenous access should be established with large-bore catheters. Preoperative administration of diphenhydramine and/or a corticosteroid may help reduce an anaphylactic reaction to spillage of cyst contents. In the event of anaphylactic shock, rapid administration of fluids, epinephrine, additional corticosteroids, and diphenhydramine will require the presence of the large-bore intravenous catheters.

The anesthetist should anticipate large fluid shifts, large volumes of fluid administration, and the potential loss of large volumes of blood, which are also reasons to use large-bore intravenous catheters.

Hydatidiform Mole

Definition

Hydatidiform mole encompasses several conditions, including complete and partial moles, placental site trophoblastic tumors, choriocarcinomas, and invasive moles. Complete moles are devoid of any fetal tissue and the chorionic villi develop grapelike (hydatiform) swelling. In addition, trophoblastic hyperplasia is present. Hydatidiform mole is also called gestational trophoblastic disease.

Incidence

The incidence of hydatidiform mole in Western countries is 1:1000 to 1:1500 pregnancies; in Asia it is 1:120 pregnancies.

Etiology

Hydatidiform mole results from the transfer of *only* paternal chromosomes, either by single spermatic fertilization of an anucleate ovum, whereupon the paternal DNA replicates, or the fertilization of an ovum by two sperm. The chorionic villi subsequently develop grapelike, or hydatiform swelling.

Signs and Symptoms

- Absent fetal heart tones
- Hyperemesis
- Hyperthyroidism
- Preeclampsia
- Tachycardia
- Tremor
- Uterine enlargement greater than normal for estimated gestational age
- Uterine enlargement smaller than normal for estimated gestational age
- Warm skin

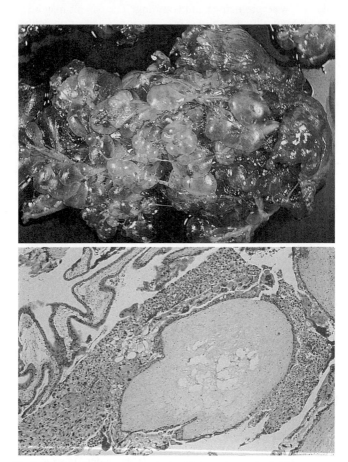

Hydatidiform Mole. Complete hydatidiform mole. Nearly all villi are
enlarged and are interconnected by thin nonedematous cordlike structures.
(*From Damjanov I, Linder J:* Pathology: A Color Atlas, *St Louis, 2000, Mosby.*)

Medical Management

Vaginal bleeding is the most common presenting symptom, followed by severe nausea and vomiting. The patient may be hemodynamically unstable on presentation. The first objective is to stabilize the patient via fluid administration, blood transfusion(s), and/or pharmacologic interventions. Any coagulopathy should be corrected. Hypertension should also be treated quickly.

The definitive treatment is uterine evacuation by dilation and curettage. Intravenous oxytocin is administered on dilation of the cervix and should be continued through the postoperative period to decrease the likelihood of hemorrhage. Methergine or Hemabate may be administered rather than oxytocin, particularly if response to oxytocin is deemed inadequate.

The patient may present in respiratory distress, which may stem from several causes, including trophoblastic embolism, high-output congestive heart failure resulting from anemia, and iatrogenic fluid overload.

Complications

- Anemia
- Disseminated intravascular coagulopathy (DIC)
- Hemorrhage
- High-output congestive heart failure
- Malignant trophoblastic disease
- Preeclampsia
- Respiratory distress/failure
- Trophoblastic embolism
- Uterine perforation

Anesthesia Implications

The patient with hydatiform mole may arrive at the OR anemic but hypovolemic, and appear as if she is hemoconcentrated. Hemoconcentration may be the result of preeclampsia or general dehydration, possibly from hyperemesis. Intravenous access should be established quickly and should consist of a minimum of one large-bore catheter, although two large-bore catheters would be better. Heart rate and blood pressure should be measured to help determine if the patient is in a compensated state—that is, with low-normal blood pressure accompanied by tachycardia. Skin turgor may indicate a state of dehydration. It may be appropriate to administer a fluid bolus and recheck the patient's fluid and electrolyte levels along with the hemoglobin and hematocrit values. These measures may help determine whether the patient is truly anemic and better indicate the need for a blood transfusion(s).

The patient who has had hyperemesis may have significant electrolyte imbalances, particularly potassium, that need to be treated in addition to the dehydration and anemia. Additional fluid boluses and potassium supplements may be necessary.

The presence of preeclampsia must be confirmed or ruled out. If present, preeclampsia becomes the primary focus. The patient with preeclampsia should receive the "full complement" of invasive monitoring: central venous catheter, pulmonary artery catheter, and arterial pressure monitoring, along with pharmacotherapy to stabilize, reduce, and control the patient's blood pressure.

Hemorrhage may be the precipitating factor that brings the patient to the OR. The hemorrhaging will likely worsen with the onset of uterine relaxation. Since all volatile anesthetic agents produce some degree of uterine relaxation, exacerbation of the patient's hemorrhaging is relatively inevitable. An inhalational anesthetic should be used in the lowest concentration feasible to maintain general anesthesia. Because of the uterine relaxation that may result from inhalational agents, the anesthetist may opt to employ total intravenous anesthesia (TIVA). The anesthetist, in a coordinated effort with the gynecologist, may need to infuse oxytocin to help reduce blood loss regardless of which technique is employed, TIVA or inhalational anesthesia. Care should be taken not to infuse the oxytocin too rapidly because it can produce significant hypotension that may last 3 to 5 minutes without response to vasopressors. Oxytocin is contraindicated in the patient with signs and symptoms of preeclampsia.

Hydrocephalus

Definition

Hydrocephalus is a disturbance or interruption of the formation, flow, or absorption of cerebrospinal fluid. All types of hydrocephalus culminate in increased volume of fluid within the central nervous system's relatively closed spaces.

Types of Hydrocephalus	
• Arrested	• Noncommunicating
• Benign external	• Normal pressure
• Communicating	• Obstructive
• Congenital	

Incidence

In the United States congenital hydrocephalus occurs at the rate of about 3:1000 live births. The frequency of acquired hydrocephalus is not documented. Internationally there are no estimates on the frequency of congenital or acquired hydrocephalus.

Etiology

Congenital Causes, Infants and Children
- Agenesis of the foramen of Monro
- Arnold-Chiari malformation (Types I and II)
- Bickers-Adams syndrome*
- Congenital toxoplasmosis
- Dandy-Walker malformation*
- Stenosis of the aqueduct of Sylvius

Acquired Causes, Infants and Children
- Iatrogenic hypervitaminosis A
- Idiopathic
- Increased venous sinus pressure
- Infections (meningitis, cysticercosis)
- Intraventricular hemorrhage
- Mass lesions

*See Appendix G: Rare Syndromes.

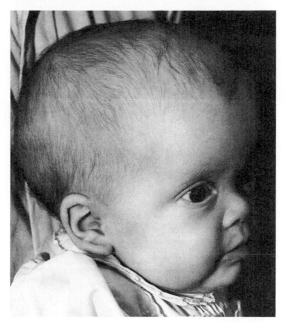

Hydrocephalus. Child with enlarged head caused by hydrocephalus. *(From McLaurin DC: Pediatric Neurosurgery, ed. 2, Philadelphia, 1989, Saunders.)*

Normal Pressure Hydrocephalus and Causes, Adult
- Congenital aqueductal stenosis
- Head injury
- Idiopathic
- Meningitis
- Previous posterior fossa surgery
- Subarachnoid hemorrhage
- Tumor

Signs and Symptoms

Manifestations are influenced by the following five factors:
1. Cause
2. Duration
3. Obstruction location
4. Patient age
5. Rapidity of onset

Infant
- Irritability
- Poor feeding
- Reduced activity
- Vomiting

Child
- Blurred vision
- Difficulty walking
- Double vision
- Drowsiness
- Headaches
- Neck pain
- Slowing mental capacity
- Spasticity
- Stunted growth or sexual maturation
- Vomiting

Adult
- Blurred vision
- Cognitive deterioration
- Difficulty walking
- Double vision
- Drowsiness
- Headaches
- Incontinence
- Nausea
- Neck pain
- Vomiting

Normal Pressure Hydrocephalus
- Aggression
- Dementia
- Gait disturbances
- Parkinson-like symptoms
- Seizures
- Urinary incontinence

Medical Management

Medical interventions are used to delay surgical intervention and are not typically effective in the long-term management of hydrocephalus. Medical intervention may work well in a preterm infant who has posthemorrhagic hydrocephalus, but not acute hydrocephalus, by fostering normal tissue development and eventual spontaneous resumption of normal cerebrospinal fluid (CSF) absorption. Medication may be used to either decrease CSF production by the choroid plexus or to increase the reabsorption of CSF that is produced.

Definitive treatment for hydrocephalus is surgical intervention, including the placement of shunts. Five shunting methods include:

1. Ventriculoperitoneal (VP) shunt (the most common)
2. Ventriculoatrial (VA) shunt
3. Lumboperitoneal shunt (reserved only for communicating hydrocephalus, CSF fistula, or pseudotumor cerebri)
4. Torkildsen shunt (rare and only effective for acquired obstructive hydrocephalus)
5. Ventriculopleural shunt (used only when all other shunts are contraindicated)

There are alternatives to shunting, including choroid plexectomy or choroid plexus coagulation, tumor excision, stenosed aqueduct opening (has the highest morbidity and the lowest success rate), and third ventricle floor endoscopic fenestration (contraindicated in communicating hydrocephalus). Rapid-onset or acute hydrocephalus with increasing intracranial pressure is an emergency situation. Four measures that may be undertaken include:

1. Ventricular taps (infant)
2. Open ventricular drainage (child and adult)
3. Lumbar puncture in posthemorrhagic and postmeningitic hydrocephalus
4. VP or VA shunt procedure

Complications

- Chronic papilledema
- Cognitive dysfunction
- Gait disturbances
- Incontinence
- Occlusion of posterior cerebral arteries
- Optic chiasm compression due to third ventricle dilation
- Visual disturbances

Specific to Medical Treatment
- Electrolyte imbalance
- Metabolic acidosis

Specific to Surgical Intervention

- Abdominal organ perforation
- Arachnoiditis
- CSF ascites
- Endocarditis
- Extraneural metastasis
- Hardware erosion
- Increased(ing) intracranial pressure
- Infection
- Inguinal hernia
- Intestinal obstruction
- Periarteritis
- Pulmonary hypertension
- Radiculopathy
- Septicemia
- Shunt embolus
- Shunt occlusion
- Subdural hematoma or hygroma
- Volvulus

Anesthesia Implications

The first consideration is the nature of the hydrocephalus. Is the case acute, subacute, or chronic? Does the patient have increased intracranial pressure (ICP)? Acute hydrocephalus with signs of increased(ing) ICP is an emergency situation. The patient should be induced, intubated, and hyperventilated fairly quickly. Because succinylcholine produces an increase in the ICP, it should be avoided in favor of a fast-onset, nondepolarizing muscle relaxant. Succinylcholine should also be omitted if the patient is being treated in the short term with either acetazolamide or furosemide or both, because of the potential hypokalemia that either or both can produce.

The anesthetist must be ever mindful of the importance of monitoring the patient's cerebral perfusion pressure (CPP). Induction, particularly in the emergent situation above, must be accomplished in such a manner as to minimize the drop in the patient's mean arterial pressure (MAP).

Remember: CPP = MAP − ICP

Premedication, although not specifically contraindicated in the patient with hydrocephalus, must be undertaken judiciously to avoid oversedation, hypoventilation, hypoxia, hypercarbia, increased cerebral blood volume, and elevation of the patient's ICP.

   The anesthetist should provide mild hyperventilation during induction and during the initial phase of the surgical intervention to "relax" the brain—reduce the level of CO_2 and constrict the cerebral blood vessels. As part of this goal, the anesthetist may need to administer an osmotic diuretic to reduce the circulating volume and further lower the cerebral blood volume. Administering such a medication too rapidly may induce a seizure, systemic hypotension, pulmonary hypertension, and congestive heart failure, among other untoward actions.

H

Incontinentia Pigmenti

Definition

Incontinentia pigmenti is a rare, X-linked, dominant inherited disorder involving skin pigmentation. Melanin is lost from the basal cells of the epidermis and collects in the dermis as free pigment or as aggregates of melanophages. Incontinentia pigmenti is also known as Bloch-Sulzberger syndrome.

Incidence

The incidence of incontinentia pigmenti is 1:40,000. The disorder is more common among Caucasian populations than other races. It affects females almost exclusively. Male fetuses typically expire in utero, although some do survive. The overall male to female ratio is 1:37.

Etiology

Almost all cases of incontinentia pigmenti occur as the result of a deletion in the NEMO gene; about half are spontaneous mutations.

Signs and Symptoms

Four Stages of Skin Change

1. Vesicular stage: linear vesicles; pustules; bullae with erythema along the lines of Blaschko; present at birth
2. Verrucous stage: warty; keratotic papules and plaques; occurs between 2 and 8 weeks of age
3. Hyperpigmentation stage: macular hyperpigmentation in a swirl pattern along the lines of Blaschko; changes often involve nipples, axilla, and groin; occurs between 12 and 40 weeks of age
4. Hypopigmentation stage: streaks and/or patches of hypopigmentation along with cutaneous atrophy; onset in infancy remaining throughout adulthood

Central Nervous System (10% to 40% of Patients)

- Ataxia
- Hyperactivity
- Mental retardation
- Microcephaly
- Seizures
- Spasticity
- Stroke

Ocular Changes

- Band keratopathy
- Blue sclera
- Cataracts
- Congenital glaucoma
- Exudative retinal detachment
- Foveal hypoplasia
- Leukocoria
- Microphthalmia
- Optic atrophy
- Retinal pigmentary changes
- Retrolental mass formation
- Strabismus

Skeletal/Structural (≈14% of Patients)

- Acheiria
- Ear abnormalities
- Extra ribs
- Hemivertebrae
- Scoliosis
- Skull deformities
- Somatic asymmetry
- Spina bifida
- Syndactyly

Teeth and Jaw Changes (65% to 90% of Patients)

- Delayed eruption
- Hypodontia
- Microdontia
- Micrognathia
- Prognathia
- Round, conical, or peg-shaped teeth

Medical Management

Currently there is no specific treatment available for incontinentia pigmenti. Lesions of stage 1 (vesicular) skin changes should be kept clean and as undisturbed as possible. Frequent, meticulous dental care and hygiene are very important.

Complications

- Blindness or reduced visual acuity due to ophthalmic changes
- Mental retardation (seen predominantly in patients with structural brain deformity or ischemic brain injury)

- Secondary bacterial infection during vesicular stage (rare)
- Seizures (seen predominately in patients with structural brain deformity or ischemic brain injury)

Anesthesia Implications

The predominance of dental and jaw abnormalities associated with incontinentia pigmenti constitutes a significant portion of anesthesia concerns. The dental abnormalities predispose the patient to potential dental injury during direct laryngoscopy. Extra care should be taken with airway manipulation. Micrognathia or prognathia in a patient with incontinentia pigmenti can have a significant impact on the anesthetist's ability to secure the airway. A difficult airway cart with a fiberoptic bronchoscope should be immediately available in the event that attempts via direct laryngoscopy prove unsuccessful. It may be more prudent, based on the situation revealed by the preoperative physical examination combined with the anesthetist's experience and skill level, to forgo direct laryngoscopy in favor of the fiberoptic approach. The level of sedation provided by the anesthetist to facilitate the fiberoptic intubation will be dictated, in large part, by the age—chronologic and/or mental development—of the patient.

Frequently the patient with incontinentia pigmenti is blind, thus requiring more detailed explanations and direction for transfer to the operating room bed. The anesthetist should tailor the depth of explanation to the patient by the patient's age, both chronologic and developmental.

The patient with associated spastic paralysis should not receive succinylcholine to facilitate intubation. The patient with a high-level spinal cord lesion is more likely to develop autonomic hyperreflexia.

Choice of anesthetic technique, general versus regional, will be predicated on the patient's age (as described above) and any associated anomalies. The very young patient or one mentally challenged may best be served by choosing general anesthesia. General anesthesia may also be the better choice for the patient with associated spinal cord lesions.

Kearns-Sayre Syndrome

Definition

Kearns-Sayre syndrome is a very rare mitochondrial DNA disorder in which there is marked heterogenicity along with various inheritance patterns. It is distinguished by three features: (1) onset before 20 years of age; (2) a chronic, progressive external ophthalmoplegia; and (3) pigmentary degeneration of the retina.

Incidence

As of 1992, a total of 226 cases of Kearns-Sayre syndrome have been documented in all of medical literature. There is no observed predilection with regard to race or gender.

Etiology

Kearns-Sayre syndrome occurs as the result of mitochondrial DNA (mtDNA) deletions that produce a particular, peculiar phenotype. Most of the mtDNA deletions in this disorder are sporadic but occur most commonly between positions 8469 and 13147.

Signs and Symptoms

- Ataxia
- Cardiac conduction defects
- Cardiomyopathy
- Diabetes mellitus
- Fanconi syndrome (see p. 132)
- Hypothyroidism
- Lactic acidosis
- Muscle weakness
- Ophthalmoplegia
- Peripheral neuropathy
- Pigmentary retinopathy
- Ptosis
- Ragged, red fibers on muscle biopsy
- Sensorineural hearing loss
- Short stature
- Sideroblastic anemia

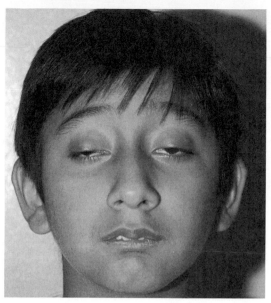

Kearns-Sayre Syndrome. In this patient, note the arching of the brows in an effort to lift the eyelids to reduce the ptosis. *(From Swartz MH: Textbook of Physical Diagnosis: History and Examination, cd. 5, Philadelphia, 2006, Saunders.)*

Medical Management

Therapy to modify (cure) Kearns-Sayre syndrome does not currently exist. Ongoing research is directed at inhibiting replication of the mutant mtDNA or developing a way to encourage replication of wild-type mtDNA (nonmutated mtDNA).

True medical management consists of treatment of specific physiologic problems that may arise in association with the mtDNA mutation: insulin may be required to treat diabetes mellitus; a pacemaker may need to be inserted to treat the development of a harmful heart block; exercise routines may be established to manage myopathy(ies). Various vitamin supplements along with coenzyme Q_{10} have demonstrated beneficial effects in individual situations. Death commonly occurs in the third or fourth decade of life.

Complications

- Deterioration of a wide range of observed signs and symptoms
- Heart block

Anesthesia Implications

The patient with an mtDNA disorder such as Kearns-Sayre syndrome is at greater risk for adverse events, including neurologic status deterioration, stroke, seizures, coma, respiratory failure, dysrhythmias, and death. Because of the increased risk for adverse anesthetic outcomes, no particular technique can be distinguished as the "best."

The patient with an mtDNA disorder is potentially more susceptible to malignant hyperthermia (MH) and/or myasthenia-like symptoms. In particular, the patient demonstrates greater sensitivity to nondepolarizing neuromuscular blocking agents. Because of the greater potential for MH, it is recommended that MH precautions be employed.

Succinylcholine should be avoided as well as other known MH triggers such as volatile inhalational agents. Total intravenous anesthesia may be a better choice for the patient with Kearns-Sayre syndrome.

Both the anesthetist and the patient should be prepared for the possibility that mechanical ventilatory support may need to be extended into the postoperative period because of residual muscle weakness. Admission to the intensive care unit should be arranged preoperatively so that close monitoring of the patient's ventilatory status can continue without undue interruption.

Because of the patient's propensity for lactic acidosis and because diabetes mellitus occurs frequently with this syndrome, the choice of intravenous fluid is important. To decrease the lactate load, lactated Ringer's solution should not be used. The blood glucose level should be monitored frequently during surgery. Incorporation of glucose-containing solutions may be necessary. Insertion of an arterial pressure catheter may be prudent to facilitate the frequent blood sampling for glucose monitoring, serum lactate concentrations, and/or blood gas analysis.

A patient with an mtDNA disorder usually has poor tolerance for long periods of fasting. Typically the patient has
become accustomed to eating frequent, small meals, and an
accelerated intake schedule may be difficult to resolve. A possible scenario could be to allow intake of clear liquids containing
some calories up to 2 hours preoperatively, with elimination of
solid food occurring 8 hours before the surgery and anesthesia.
Scheduling the patient's surgery as the first case of the day will
help facilitate patient compliance.

K

Klippel-Feil Syndrome

Definition

Klippel-Feil syndrome is a rare congenital disorder in which any two of the seven cervical vertebrae are absent or fused, resulting in a short neck with limited range of motion.

Classification of Klippel-Feil Syndrome	
Type I	Massive fusion of the cervical spine
Type II	Fusion of one or two cervical interspaces
Type III	Thoracic and/or lumbar spine anomalies in conjunction with Type I or II

Incidence

The true incidence of Klippel-Feil syndrome is not known.

Etiology

The true etiology of Klippel-Feil syndrome is not fully understood. There are various suggestions as to the etiology of this malady, including congenital failure of segmentation of the cervical vertebrae, which results from failure of segmentation of cervical somites during the third through eighth weeks of gestation. Some have suggested the occurrence of some manner of global fetal insult, whereas others suggest the malady may be caused by some manner of vascular disruption.

Signs and Symptoms

For anomalies, see box below.

Anomalies Associated with Klippel-Feil Syndrome	
• Brainstem anomalies	• Renal disease (horseshoe kidney, renal ectopia, bilateral tubular ectasia, hydronephrosis, absent kidney)
• Congenital heart disorder (most commonly ventricular septal defect)	
• Congenital scoliosis	
• Craniosynostosis	• Sprengel's deformity (elevation of scapula)
• Dyskinesia	

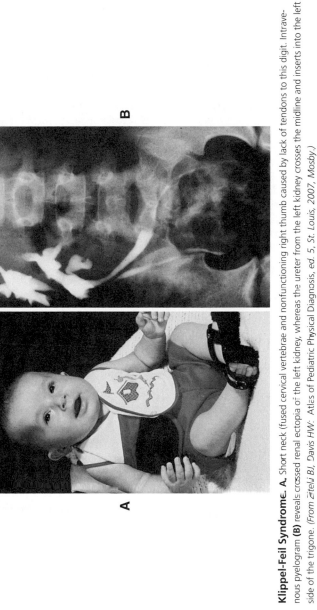

Klippel-Feil Syndrome. A, Short neck (fused cervical vertebrae and nonfunctioning right thumb caused by lack of tendons to this digit. Intravenous pyelogram **(B)** reveals crossed renal ectopia of the left kidney, whereas the ureter from the left kidney crosses the midline and inserts into the left side of the trigone. (*From Zitelli BJ, Davis HW:* Atlas of Pediatric Physical Diagnosis, *ed. 5, St. Louis, 2007, Mosby.*)

K

- Abnormal hand position
- Ataxia
- Blurred vision
- Bruxism
- Decreased cervical range of motion (rotational loss)
- Difficulty swallowing
- Disturbed phonation
- Dizziness
- Duane syndrome (eye contracture)
- Facial asymmetry
- Facial nerve palsy
- Headache
- Hearing loss
- Hydrocephalus
- Hypermobility of unaffected interspaces
- Hypoplastic thumb
- Lateral rectus palsy
- Low hairline
- Micrognathia
- Neck webbing
- Nystagmus
- Oligodontia of deciduous permanent teeth
- Palatal clefts
- Ptosis
- Restrictive mouth opening
- Short neck
- Supernumerary digits
- Syndactyly
- Temporomandibular joint dysfunction
- Torticollis
- Upper extremity hypoplasia

Medical Management

Because of instability of the cervical spine, quadriplegia and even death can occur as the result of relatively minor trauma. The patient is therefore cautioned to strictly avoid contact sports, particularly those that place the neck at particular risk. Mechanical symptoms may be treated with a cervical collar, analgesics, nonsteroidal anti-inflammatory drugs, or even judicial application of cervical traction.

Further medical treatment regimens may be indicated for associated systemic anomalies. Treatment regimens should involve a medical specialist for that particular anomaly (e.g., cardiologist, nephrologist, urologist). Surgical intervention(s) may be indicated for several reasons, such as neurologic deficits, persistent pain, and spinal stenosis.

Complications

- Ataxia
- Death
- Quadriplegia
- Seizures
- Spinal cord compression
- Syncope

Anesthesia Implications

Before anesthesia the patient should undergo a thorough series of x-rays of the head and neck. A complete evaluation of any associated systemic anomaly must be completed as well. Clinical manifestations may result either from compression of the cervical spine, the pons, or medulla or from stretching of cranial nerves. Basilar artery compromise may occur as the result of sudden neck rotation and syncope may ensue.

One of the highest priorities for the anesthetist is positioning, more specifically positioning of the patient's head and neck throughout anesthesia care. The patient's head and neck should be maintained in neutral alignment at all times. Quadriplegia and death have been reported with even minor trauma in patients with Klippel-Feil syndrome. The patient should demonstrate his or her neck range of motion to delineate any resulting symptoms that may arise.

The patient scheduled for general anesthesia may prove difficult to intubate because of the decreased neck range of motion. The anesthetist, in conjunction with the patient, must decide preoperatively whether the intubation will be performed with the patient awake or asleep. The advantage of an awake attempt would be the patient's ability to communicate the onset of any problematic sequelae during the intubation attempt. Placing the patient in the "sniffing" position for intubation may actually cause harm. To maintain neutral alignment it may be necessary to enlist the aid of another anesthetist to apply gentle cervical traction during laryngoscopy. The anesthetist must abort or abandon direct laryngoscopy if the patient's head and neck cannot be maintained in neutral alignment throughout the intubation attempt. It may be necessary to forgo direct laryngoscopy in favor of the fiberoptic bronchoscopic direct visualization.

For either intubation attempt, the oropharynx should be very well anesthetized to negate the patient's gag reflex. The vocal cords should be anesthetized using local anesthetic injected via the cricothyroid membrane. Some sedation would be appropriate for this procedure, but the anesthetist should be mindful of the great need for patient cooperation and communication throughout this attempt. Once the airway is secured, the patient may receive the scheduled general anesthetic induction medication doses. Muscle relaxation should be achieved using nondepolarizing muscle relaxants. As with the intubation, patient positioning for the surgical procedure must primarily focus on maintaining neutral axial alignment of the head and neck.

Emergence and extubation for the patient require good communication among anesthetist, patient, and surgeon. Consensus should be obtained before anesthesia concerning this process. The optimal situation is for the patient to be fully in control of airway reflexes and not coughing or "bucking" on the endotracheal tube, thus risking potentially fatal sequelae. On the other hand, extubating the relatively deeply anesthe-tized patient presents the risk of airway obstruction in the patient with a potentially difficult airway.

Regional anesthesia, specifically continuous subarachnoid anesthesia, has been reported to be successful. Once again, good communication is paramount. Intravenous sedation for anxiolysis may be given with the regional anesthetic, but such administration must be judicious— even "stingy"— to avert airway obstruction. Should airway obstruction occur, the anes-thetist must take great care while alleviating that obstruction not to induce extreme movement of the patient's neck, par-ticularly axial rotation, and so avoid very deleterious sequelae.

Long QT Syndrome

Definition

Long QT syndrome (LQTS) is prolonged duration of the QT interval in the cardiac cycle. This syndrome can be congenital or acquired. The congenital form may or may not be accompanied by deafness. Both forms have a propensity for ventricular dysrhythmias, which in turn may lead to unstable dysrhythmias (e.g., torsades de pointes, ventricular fibrillation), syncope, cardiac arrest, and/or sudden death.

Incidence

The true incidence of LQTS is difficult to estimate. It can be acquired or congenital, as a result of genetic mutations; approximately 10% to 15% of gene mutation carriers have normal QT_C duration. Overall, LQTS may occur as frequently as 1:3000 to 1:5000.

Etiology

The congenital form of LQTS is the result of the mutation of cardiac ion channel genes. Thus far six chromosomal mutation locations and five specific genes have been identified. There are six variants of LQTS associated with Romano-Ward syndrome and two variants associated with Jervell and Lange-Nielsen syndrome. The prolongation of the QT interval occurs when the myocardial cells become overloaded with positively charged ions during the process of ventricular repolarization. This prolongation predisposes the patient to unstable ventricular dysrhythmias, particularly torsades de pointes, ventricular fibrillation, and sudden cardiac death. The appearance of ventricular dysrhythmias may be precipitated by any of a large number of adrenergic stimuli, including exercise, emotion, loud noises, atnd startle, but may occur spontaneously without preceding conditions or triggers. As a result, the patient with LQTS should be generally discouraged from participation in competitive sports.

LQTS can be acquired as a result of ingestion of various medications. The complete list of medications that may produce LQTS and/or an incidence of torsades de pointes is too large to be included in this volume, but it includes

amiodarone, erythromycin, methadone, procainamide, and
quinidine. A complete list of the medications can be found at
www.qtdrugs.org/medical-pros/drug-lists/list-01.cfm.

Signs and Symptoms

- Aborted cardiac arrest
- Congenital deafness
- Family history of sudden cardiac death (especially at a young age)
- Notched T-wave in three leads
- Slow heart rate for patient age
- Sudden death
- Syncope
- Torsades de pointes
- T-wave alternans

Medical Management

The pharmacologic choice for management of LQTS is the use
of a β blocker. β Blockers reduce the risk of cardiac dysrhythmia
by blocking the adrenergic response. Until recently β blockers
have been given in large doses (e.g., propranolol, 3 mg/kg/day).
Current data suggest that a smaller dose may deliver protective
effects similar to that observed with the larger doses. The most
commonly used β blockers are propranolol and nadolol, although
atenolol and metoprolol are also frequently prescribed. β Blockade is *not* a curative treatment. About 70% of LQTS patients
are effectively treated (i.e., cardiac events are prevented) with
β blockers; however, about 30% may still experience a cardiac
event. Gene-specific therapy is not presently available to treat the
alteration or mutations to the relevant ion channel(s).

A patient deemed to be at greatest risk for a cardiac event
may benefit from having a cardioverter-defibrillator implanted.
A higher risk patient is defined as one who has experienced an
aborted cardiac arrest, has recurrent cardiac events despite conventional pharmacologic therapy, or uses β blockers combined
with a cardiac pacemaker and/or stellectomy. Left cervicotho-
racic stellectomy may be used as an antiadrenergic therapy in a
high-risk LQTS patient.

Complications

- Cardiac arrest
- Neurologic deficits (after an aborted cardiac arrest)
- Sudden death

- Torsades de pointes
- Ventricular fibrillation

Anesthesia Implications

First and foremost, the patient with LQTS *must* continue the usual oral dose of β blocking medication(s) on the operative day. Anxiety should be treated prophylactically with a preoperative anxiolytic medication, "erring" on the larger end of the dosage range. To minimize adrenergic stimulation, the patient should ideally be deeply anesthetized before any attempt at direct laryngoscopy. The anesthetic course should be charted with every effort directed at minimizing adrenergic stimulation. The technique should rely fairly heavily on opioid administration to blunt or suppress adrenergic response to noxious stimulation. Nitrous oxide should not be used because of its inherent mild sympathetic stimulation. For this same reason, desflurane should not be the volatile agent chosen for the maintenance of general anesthesia. Epinephrine should be avoided, whether in conjunction with regional anesthesia or for treatment of hypotension or bradycardia. Isoflurane and sevoflurane are each known to prolong the QT interval and are best avoided; halothane reduces the QT interval and may be used if it is available. Propofol also reduces the QT interval as well as QT dispersion. Total intravenous anesthesia (TIVA) may be the most appropriate choice for the patient with LQTS. At the conclusion of surgery it may be appropriate to extubate the patient while he or she is still relatively deeply anesthetized—unless there are contraindications such as gastroesophageal reflux disease (GERD) or morbid obesity—to minimize any anxiety and/or adrenergic stimulation during the emergence process. For longer, more extensive surgical procedures, a supplemental infusion of a β blocker may be indicated. This infusion should be continued into the postanesthesia care phase before being tapered to discontinuation. Pain must be adequately controlled postoperatively, along with any nausea or vomiting.

Lown-Ganong-Levine Syndrome

Definition

Lown-Ganong-Levine (LGL) syndrome is a preexcitation syndrome producing supraventricular tachycardia that is neither atrial fibrillation nor atrial flutter. This syndrome is characterized by a short P-R interval (<20 milliseconds) and normal QRS complexes.

Incidence

The incidence of LGL syndrome is estimated to be approximately 0.5% worldwide.

Etiology

Some evidence suggests that LGL is a hereditary condition in some families. No definitive structural/anatomic anomaly has been identified as yet. Many experts believe that LGL is not a syndrome itself, but a manifestation of any of several maladies.

Signs and Symptoms

- Chest pain
- Hypotension
- Lightheadedness
- Palpitations
- Paroxysmal tachycardia
- Shortness of breath

Medical Management

There is no medical treatment specifically for LGL syndrome. Interventions are directed at identifying and resolving the cause of the tachycardia. When episodes produce symptoms, hospitalization is indicated, with the priority being to gain control of the patient's ventricular heart rate. Immediate measures include Valsalva maneuver and/or carotid massage if there are no carotid bruits. Failure of these measures to interrupt the tachydysrhythmia may indicate the need to administer adenosine during continuous electrocardiography monitoring and recording. Treatment of the episodic paroxysmal supraventricular tachycardia may be undertaken on an outpatient basis.

Pharmacologic treatment options include β-blocking medications, calcium channel–blocking medications, and digoxin. In the most extreme conditions/scenarios, radiofrequency ablation of either the AV node or bundle of His may be indicated. After successful pathway ablation, a pacemaker must be implanted.

Complications

Any complications are attributable to the underlying condition.

Anesthesia Implications

Frequently the patient with LGL presents for accessory pathway ablation. As such, pharmacologic interventions are usually stopped to aid in inducing a tachydysrhythmia. The patient is pharmacologically unprotected. Anxiolysis is important to lessen the chance of inciting a tachydysrhythmia in relatively uncontrolled surroundings, such as the patient's room, the elevator, and/or the anesthesia holding room. Relatively heavy premedication is most helpful in achieving the desired degree of anxiolysis. If a tachydysrhythmia occurs, it may be controlled using very short-acting agents, such as esmolol or adenosine.

L

Ludwig's Angina

Definition

Ludwig's angina is cellulitis of the mouth floor. It expands very rapidly and can spread to other areas of the body, such as the mediastinum or the coccyx, via the myriad tissue planes found within the neck. Ludwig's angina is potentially fatal.

Incidence

Currently there is no accurate estimate for the frequency at which this severe form of cellulitis occurs.

Etiology

For 100 years after the original description, Ludwig's angina was generally viewed as a complication of a local anesthetic agent infiltration given for extraction of mandibular molars. The actual pathogenesis is the extension and expansion of a dental abscess into the submandibular space(s). Even today, the majority of Ludwig's angina cases are initiated by an odontogenic source.

Possible Sources of Ludwig's Angina	
• Brachial cleft anomalies	• Necrosis and suppuration of a malignant cervical lymph node or mass
• Cervical lymphadenitis	
• Compound mandibular fracture	
• Dental abscesses/infections	• Oral surgical procedures
• Foreign body aspiration	• Otitis media
• Infected malignancy	• Penetrating trauma to the oral cavity pharynx
• IV drug use/abuse	
• Lymphalocele	• Salivary gland infection/obstruction
• Mastoiditis with apicitis of the petrous part of the temporal bone and Bezold's abscess (abscess in the neck with pus tracts deep to the superior portion of the sternocleidomastoid muscle and along the posterior belly of the digastric muscle)	• Sialadenitis
	• Thyroiditis
	• Tonsillar and pharyngeal infections

L

Infectious Organisms Associated with Ludwig's Angina

- *Bacteroides melaninogenicus*
- *Bacteroides oralis*
- *Escherichia coli*
- *Fusobacterium nucleatum*
- *Hemophilus influenzae*
- Peptostreptococcus species
- Pseudomonas species
- Spirochaeta species
- *Staphylococcus aureus*
- *Streptococcus pneumoniae*
- *Streptococcus pyogenes*
- *Streptococcus viridans*

Signs and Symptoms

- Difficulty breathing
- Dysphonia
- Edema of neck, tongue, and the submandibular region
- Fear
- Increased salivation
- Pain
- Protruding tongue
- Trismus

Medical Management

The highest priority for care of a patient with Ludwig's angina is to ensure a patent airway. This form of cellulitis spreads/expands quite rapidly. Despite the numerous fascial planes within the neck, the expansion of the inflammatory edema is limited by the mandible, hyoid bone, and superficial layer of the deep cervical fascia. As a result, the tongue and mouth floor may be displaced in a superior and posterior direction. The lingual displacement and frequent laryngeal edema can quickly overrun and completely occlude the airway, culminating in death by asphyxiation. Direct laryngoscopy for endotracheal intubation may be extremely difficult or impossible. It may quickly become necessary to have the airway secured surgically via tracheostomy. Such a decision must be made very rapidly to avert fatal sequelae.

If this infectious process has progressed to the point that the airway must be secured by surgical means, the submandibular region and other areas need to be explored. The areas should be incised, irrigated, and drained. Wound cultures should be obtained to identify the causative organism and determine the most appropriate antibiotic to treat the infection. Parenteral antibiotics should be administered until the patient has been afebrile for at least 48 hours. Before antibiotics were available, the mortality with this disease was more than 50%. Early diagnosis and aggressive antibiotic therapy has reduced mortality to less than 2%.

Complications

- Airway obstruction
- Aspiration
- Carotid artery erosion/ rupture
- Cranial nerve dysfunction
- Grisel syndrome
- Innominate artery rupture
- Mandibular osteomyelitis
- Mediastinal abscess
- Mediastinitis
- Necrotizing fasciitis
- Osteomyelitis (cervical)
- Pericardial effusion
- Pleural effusion
- Pneumothorax
- Septic emboli
- Septic shock
- Subphrenic abscess
- Thrombosis of internal jugular

Anesthesia Implications

Airway management is the most critical factor. It may be most appropriate and prudent to secure the patient's airway surgically via awake tracheostomy, using local anesthetic infiltration and minimal or no sedation. Intravenous induction may cause near-instantaneous loss of the patient's airway. Awake fiberoptic intubation may be preferable to direct laryngoscopy. Instrumentation of the patient's airway should be held to a minimum because of the additional airway edema that may be evoked by the manipulation. Sedation must be kept at a minimum for the awake fiberoptic attempt. Because of a high potential for continued further expansion of the airway edema, an armored endotracheal tube may be the most appropriate choice to secure the patient's airway.

It would be wise to keep the patient ventilated by whatever method has been successful—nasotracheal or orotracheal intubation or tracheostomy—and ensure that the patient is sedated and comfortable. Repeated trips to the operating room may be necessary for serial incision and drainage of the infected area. It is important to remember that it will take time for the intravenous antibiotic therapy to become optimally effective.

Lymphangioleiomyomatosis

Definition

Lymphangioleiomyomatosis (LAM) affects women during the childbearing years. It is characterized by proliferation of smooth muscle phenotypic neoplastic cells in the lungs, kidneys, and axial lymphatics. The proliferation results in cystic destruction of the lung with progressive pulmonary dysfunction and abdominal tumors.

Incidence

The incidence of LAM is unknown. More than 500 cases had been documented in the United States as of 2006.

Etiology

The etiology of LAM is unknown. The disease occurs predominately in premenopausal women and seems to be exacerbated by elevated estrogen states, suggesting that female hormones may have a prominent role in the cause.

Signs and Symptoms

- Chest pain
- Chylothorax
- Chylous ascites
- Chyluria (chyle in the urine)
- Cough
- Dyspnea
- Lymphedema
- Pleural effusions
- Pneumoperitoneum
- Pneumothorax(-aces)

Medical Management

Generalized medical care of the patient with LAM is directed toward treatment of specific symptoms.

Pleural effusions may be treated with chemical pleurodesis or surgical obliteration of the pleural space. Pulmonary dysfunction is treated with good, generalized pulmonary care incorporating bronchodilators and supplemental oxygen. In extreme circumstances, lung transplantation may be considered.

Ascites may be treated with paracentesis to remove the fluid.

Hormonal manipulation has been advocated. Medroxyprogesterone and gonadotropin-releasing hormone agonists have been advocated, but case reports are inconclusive. More recent experimental drug therapies include sirolimus, doxycycline, and octreotide.

Complications

- Benign metastasizing leiomyoma
- Bronchiolitis
- Diffuse pulmonary lymphangiomatosis
- Eosinophilic granuloma
- Interstitial pulmonary fibrosis
- Leiomyosarcoma
- Lymphangiomas
- Pleural effusion(s)
- Pneumothorax
- Pulmonary lymphangiectasis
- Smooth muscle cell proliferation in the lung
- Tuberous sclerosis

Anesthesia Implications

Malnutrition and immunocompromise are two concerns in the patient with LAM presenting to the OR. Malnutrition carries with it a host of associated problems, including electrolyte imbalances, low levels of serum proteins, lipid imbalances, altered energy reserves, altered protein synthesis, myocardial dysfunction, and loss of muscle strength. Preoperative laboratory studies must necessarily concentrate on evaluating levels of electrolytes, serum proteins, and glucose as well as bleeding times (PT, PTT, and bleeding time) to give the anesthetist an opportunity to initiate corrective measures. Sodium and potassium imbalances may require intravenous supplementation along with infusion of solutions containing 5% albumin and glucose. Hypolipidemia may be treated with a lipid infusion. The low level of serum proteins and altered protein synthesis may adversely affect the patient's ability to synthesize necessary clotting factors. The patient may require infusion(s) of fresh frozen plasma to supplement the serum proteins and to temporarily enhance the patient's clotting factors. As a result of the altered protein synthesis and the subsequent alteration in clotting factors, the anesthetist should anticipate greater blood loss than would otherwise be expected for a particular surgical procedure.

The patient's state or degree of malnutrition may have a significant impact on her wound healing ability. If possible, elective surgery should be postponed to allow for several days of hyperalimentation to improve her nutritional state.

The degree of immunosuppression may be tied to the patient's nutritional status. Improvement of the patient's nutritional status may rebuild the patient's immune status.

LAM is associated with development of chylothorax (-thoraces). Elective surgery should be postponed until any chylothorax present can be drained and a chest tube(s) secured in place. The presence of chylothorax can produce significant atelectasis, which in turn results in ventilation/perfusion (V/Q) mismatch. This mismatch causes altered gas exchange. Thoracentesis to drain any chylothorax allows for re-expansion of the atelectatic areas but can also increase the V/Q mismatch in the affected area until the re-expanded area's ventilation improvement "catches up" with the improved perfusion. For this reason, preoperative thoracentesis should precede any surgery by several hours, if not a full day. Because of the patient's altered gas exchange, several drugs must be avoided. These drugs—which reduce hypoxic pulmonary vasoconstriction, thus worsening gas exchange and lowering arterial O_2 content—include nitroprusside, nitroglycerin, β_2-agonists, nitric oxide, and nimodipine.

LAM also affects the lung by producing a mixed obstruction/restrictive pulmonary disease. Preoperative evaluation of the patient's pulmonary status is important and must include pulmonary function tests (PFTs), arterial blood gas analysis, and chest x-ray. Intraoperative ventilation should incorporate methods to lower inspiratory pressure and allow for prolonged expiratory time, the goal being to reduce the possibility of air trapping and potential pneumothorax development. Because of the association of pneumothorax with LAM, patients who do not have a chest tube in place before anesthesia should not receive nitrous oxide as part of the anesthesia plan.

Because of the significant detrimental effects on the lungs produced by LAM, both the anesthetist and the patient should discuss the possible need for postoperative ventilatory support. The pulmonary damage, along with the malnutrition status and extensive nature of the surgery, may require that the patient remain intubated and sedated long enough to build up sufficient energy reserves to accomplish the work of breathing.

The kidneys may also be significantly altered by LAM. Blood urea nitrogen, serum creatinine, and urinary output are indicators of renal function. Fluid restrictions may be necessary when parameters indicate some degree of renal dysfunction.

Placement of an arterial pressure catheter may be prudent and convenient for the patient with LAM. This monitoring device will enable serial arterial blood gas sampling for analysis as well as assessment of fluid and electrolyte status, particularly during extensive procedures.

Lymphomatoid Granulomatosis

Definition

Lymphomatoid granulomatosis (LYG) is a rare angiodestructive, lymphoproliferative disease with significant pulmonary involvement in the form of pulmonary angiitis and granulomatosis. LYG mimics Wegner's granulomatosis (see p. 345), both in clinical and radiographic presentation.

Incidence

The frequency of LYG occurrence is not known. Males are affected more than females at a 2:1 rate.

Etiology

The true cause of LYG is not known. Recent evidence strongly suggests it is a distinct type of malignant lymphoma associated with immunosuppression. LYG is distinguished from Wegner's granulomatosis by the involvement of B-cells.

Signs and Symptoms

Definitive diagnosis of LYG is based on the histologic triad of (1) granulomatosis, (2) polymorphic lymphocytic infiltrate, and (3) angiitis. Symptoms include:

- Ataxia
- Cough
- Distal sensory neuropathy
- Dyspnea
- Erythema
- Fever
- Hemiparesis
- Hemoptysis
- Hepatomegaly
- Lymphocytic infiltration of meninges, cerebral vessels, and peripheral nerves
- Malaise
- Mental status changes
- Mononeuritis multiplex
- Patchy, painful erythematous macules, papules, and plaques
- Pneumonia
- Seizures
- Weight loss

Medical Management

A consensus for treatment of LYG has not been established. Regimens cover the spectrum from observation and occasional spontaneous remission, to prednisone administration with or without chemotherapy using agents such as cyclophosphamide. Antilymphoma regimens are employed if or when LYG progresses to a high-grade form of lymphoma, but response typically has been poor.

Localized or isolated pulmonary tumors or masses may be surgically excised and followed by chemotherapy. Interferon alfa-2b or ganciclovir are currently being used experimentally to treat LYG.

Complications

- Diabetes insipidus
- Hemoptysis
- Hemorrhage
- Mental status changes
- Mononeuropathy
- Pneumothorax
- Progressive respiratory disease
- Pulmonary infection
- Respiratory failure
- Seizures
- Sepsis
- Transformation to a high-grade lymphoma

Anesthesia Implications

The primary organs targeted by LYG are the lungs. Preoperatively the patient should receive both pulmonary function testing and arterial blood gas analysis to evaluate the extent of lung dysfunction present. Ventilatory support intraoperatively, and potentially postoperatively, will need to be individualized based on the results of the pulmonary function tests and ABGs. Postoperative ventilatory support should be discussed with the patient and/or family before surgery.

Hypoadrenalism, hypercalcemia, hypothyroidism, and hypogonadism have all been reported in association with LYG. Treatment of any of these associated conditions should be assessed and initiated before surgery and anesthesia. Supplemental steroids may be needed for patients receiving prednisone.

Neurologic sequelae of LYG do not occur very often. Typically any central nervous system (CNS) involvement results from cranial nerve palsies. Therefore the patient with LYG should undergo a good neurologic examination preoperatively.

The patient receiving chemotherapy agents, whether cyclophosphamide or vincristine, should be assessed for potential complications associated with the treatment regimen. Cyclophosphamide is associated with myelosuppression; vincristine is associated with the development of peripheral neuropathy. Any condition associated with the ongoing chemotherapy regimen should be documented during the preanesthesia interview/assessment.

L

Malignant Atrophic Papulosis

Definition

Malignant atrophic papulosis (MAP) was originally described as a variant of thromboangiitis obliterans, but was quickly recognized to be a distinct disease entity. MAP is characterized by narrowing and eventual occlusion of the lumen of small-caliber blood vessels by intimal proliferation and thrombosis. Ultimately, ischemia and infarction of the affected organ or organ system can occur. There are two distinct forms: (1) *malignant*, which can affect the heart, lungs, eyes, kidneys, pericardium, central nervous system, peripheral nervous system, and gastrointestinal system; and (2) *benign*, which is limited to the skin. Malignant atrophic papulosis is also known as Degos syndrome.

Incidence

The incidence of MAP is rare. Only about 200 cases have been reported worldwide since its initial description in 1941. Malignant atrophic papulosis is found among both sexes, predominantly in young adults and in Caucasians of Europe and North America, although cases have been documented in Japan, India, and continental Africa.

Etiology

The etiology of MAP remains unknown. There have been suggestions of autoimmune, hypersensitivity, viral, and genetic bases for this disease, but to date none have been confirmed. It is also theorized that MAP is not a single entity, but the product of several disease processes.

Signs and Symptoms

- Abdominal distention
- Abdominal pain
- Aphasia
- Bowel infarction
- Cerebral edema
- Constipation
- Constrictive pericarditis with calcification
- Decreased platelet aggregation
- Diarrhea
- Dizziness

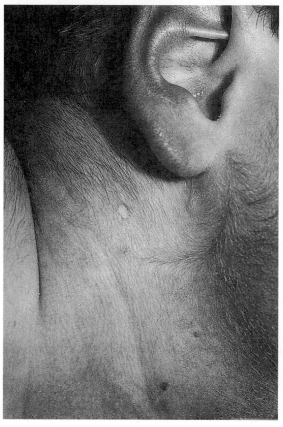

Malignant Atrophic Papulosis. Malignant atrophic papulosis, also called Degos' disease, in a patient with systemic lupus erythematosus. (*From Callen JP, et al:* Color Atlas of Dermatology, *ed 2, Philadelphia, 2000, Saunders.*)

M

- Facial or extremity paresthesias
- Fatigue
- Fistula(e)
- Gaze palsy
- Headache
- Hemiplegia
- Impaired fibrinolytic activity
- Increased intracranial pressure
- Malabsorption symptoms
- Nausea
- Paraplegia
- Peritonitis
- Pleural effusion
- Pleuritis
- Seizures
- Severe restrictive pulmonary disease
- Spastic paralysis
- Uncal herniation
- Viscus perforation
- Vomiting
- Weakness
- Weight loss

Medical Management

Since the initial description of MAP in 1941, various medications have been used to treat it, including corticosteroids, immunosuppressants, sulfonamides, tetracyclines, aspirin, dipyridamole, anticoagulants, penicillin, and interferon alfa-2a. As yet, none of those medications has demonstrated clearly any superior effectiveness in alteration of the disease process. The prognosis is that this disease is typically fatal within 2 to 3 years after the diagnosis of systemic involvement. Frequently surgical intervention is required to correct or treat gastrointestinal bleeding, perforated viscus, infarcted bowel, or possible intracranial bleeding.

Complications

- Bowel ischemia
- Cerebral infarction
- Epidural hemorrhage
- Gastrointestinal bleeding
- Intestinal perforation
- Intracerebral hemorrhage
- Neuropathy
- Pericarditis
- Peritonitis
- Pleuritis
- Spinal cord infarction
- Subdural hemorrhage

Anesthesia Implications

Because of the frequency of gastrointestinal symptoms and involvement, the patient with MAP may be either acutely or chronically dehydrated. Concomitantly the patient's electrolyte concentrations may be significantly altered from normal levels.

If the situation allows, it would be prudent to correct the fluid and electrolyte imbalances before administering anesthetia.

Both heart tones and breath sounds should be auscultated preoperatively. The patient with significant pericardial involvement may demonstrate a friction rub. Electrocardiograph and chest x-ray are also necessary to fully evaluate the patient's pulmonary and cardiac status. The anesthetist may find any manner of alterations in the electrocardiograph as a result of small infarcts over time. The presence of restrictive lung disease will require the anesthetist to reduce the peak inspiratory pressures and prolong the inspiratory time. Usually this is best accomplished by selecting the pressure-controlled ventilation option available on most late-model anesthesia machines and reducing the peak inspiratory pressure for each ventilation.

The anesthetist should also have bleeding times determined preoperatively for the patient with MAP. Both fibrinolytic activity and platelet aggregation are altered by MAP. As a result, the anesthetist should anticipate greater blood volume losses than would usually be anticipated with a procedure.

Both the peripheral and central nervous systems may be significantly altered by MAP. The anesthetist should thoroughly document any functional deficits of the peripheral nervous system preoperatively. More significant is the focus on the effects MAP may produce in the central nervous system. These effects may be quite extensive. The lesions may ultimately produce cerebral edema, which can culminate in increased intracranial pressure. The anesthetist must be astute and thorough in documenting signs and/or symptoms of increased intracranial pressure. Anesthesia-related medications should be selected with the patient's increased intracranial pressure in mind. Appropriate medications include thiopental, propofol, and narcotic analgesics. The patient should be mildly hyperventilated throughout the procedure to reduce the degree of cerebral edema. The severity of the increased intracranial pressure will be a determining factor in deciding whether to extubate the patient at the end of the procedure or to maintain mechanical ventilatory support for a period of time—an eventuality that must be thoroughly discussed with the patient and/or family preoperatively.

> ## Mallory-Weiss Tear

Definition

Mallory-Weiss tear is upper gastrointestinal bleeding produced by longitudinal mucosal lacerations (tears) at the gastroesophageal junction (cardiac sphincter). Initiation of the tear (and bleeding) can occur after a sudden rise in intragastric pressure or gastric prolapse into the esophagus.

Incidence

The incidence of Mallory-Weiss tear accounts for about 15% of all cases of upper gastrointestinal bleeding. Males are affected more than females at a rate of 2:1 to 4:1.

Etiology

Mallory-Weiss tear occurs as a result of large, rapid, transient, transmural pressure gradient generation across the area of the gastrointestinal junction. This injury may be precipitated by retching or vomiting or by violent prolapse or intussusception of the upper stomach into the lower esophagus.

Predisposing/Precipitating Factors in Mallory-Weiss Tears	
• Blunt abdominal trauma	• Primal screaming therapy
• Cardiopulmonary resuscitation	• Retching
• Coughing	• Straining
• Hiatal hernia	• Vomiting
• Hiccupping	

Signs and Symptoms

Signs and symptoms exclusive to Mallory-Weiss tears are lacking. The predominant signs and symptoms are related to the rate and degree of gastrointestinal trauma and bleeding.

- Abdominal pain
- Excessive alcohol use
- Excessive aspirin use
- Hematemesis
- Hematochezia
- Melena
- Syncope

Medical Management

Endoscopy is the definitive choice for both diagnosis and treatment modalities. The choice of endoscopic treatment depends on the endoscopist's familiarity with that technique and the equipment available to accomplish the treatment. Active bleeding is frequently treated with a contact thermal method (e.g., multipolar electrocoagulation or a heater probe), which may or may not be combined with injection of epinephrine.

Injection of epinephrine at a concentration of 1:10,000 or 1:20,000 reduces bleeding and can terminate bleeding by vasoconstriction and tamponade. Vessel sclerosis with either alcohol or polidocanol has been reported successful; however,

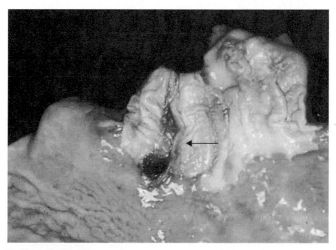

Mallory-Weiss Tear. Esophageal laceration (Mallory-Weiss tears). Gross view demonstrating longitudinal lacerations extending from esophageal mucosa into stomach mucosa *(arrow)*. (*Courtesy of Richard Harruff, MD, King County Medical Examiner's Office, Seattle, WA.*)

there are safer treatment methods available. Sclerosants introduce additional risks, including deep tissue necrosis and increased potential for perforation.

Newer treatment modalities include argon plasma coagulation, endoscopic band ligation, and endoscopic hemoclip application. All of these modalities have demonstrated efficacy in the treatment of Mallory-Weiss tears.

Patients who are refractory to endoscopic therapies or who are at higher risk for complications from endoscopic treatment modalities may receive angiotherapy via selective vasopressin infusion or embolization of the left gastric artery.

Complications

Similar to the signs and symptoms, most complications of Mallory-Weiss tear are related to the extensiveness of gastrointestinal bleeding, the patient's acuity, and any co-morbidities that may be present. Complications include:

- Death
- Esophageal perforation
- Hypovolemic shock
- Myocardial infarction
- Myocardial ischemia
- Organ ischemia and infarction secondary to angiotherapy

Anesthesia Implications

Mallory-Weiss tears are common among patients with alcohol abuse problems. They are also associated with patients who chronically ingest aspirin. In addition, this problem may occur after a bout of prolonged vomiting and/or retching. Endoscopic treatment modalities may necessitate general anesthesia to facilitate completion of the chosen modality. As such, rapid sequence induction must be implemented. Antiemetic measures should be administered perioperatively to minimize the development of nausea and vomiting and/or retching on emergence from the anesthetic. Vomiting and/or retching may result in a new esophageal injury with additional bleeding.

The patient's liver function should be evaluated preoperatively because of the strong association of this malady with ethanol abuse. Co-morbidities associated with ethanol abuse may alter the intended actions of many anesthesia-related drugs.

Chronic aspirin ingestion can produce a metabolic acidosis for which the patient may compensate with a respiratory alkalosis. The metabolic alkalosis can be exacerbated by the anesthetist if the patient is hyperventilated over the course of the surgery and duration of the anesthetic. In addition, the aspirin ingestion results in interference with platelet function and may contribute to considerable intraoperative blood loss.

M

Marfan Syndrome

Definition

Marfan syndrome is an autosomal dominant genetic defect of the connective tissue protein, fibrillin. It results in myriad clinical problems, predominately in the cardiac, musculoskeletal, and ocular systems.

Incidence

The incidence of Marfan syndrome is estimated to range from 1:5000 to 1:10,000.

Etiology

FBN 1 locus on chromosome 15 codes for the connective tissue protein, fibrillin. Mutations of the *FBN 1* locus are believed to be responsible for Marfan syndrome.

Signs and Symptoms

Cardiovascular System
- Ascending aorta dilation
- Ascending aorta dissection
- Mitral valve annulus calcification
- Mitral valve prolapse
- Pulmonary artery dilation
- Thoracic or abdominal aorta dilation or dissection

Ocular System
- Abnormally flat cornea
- Ectopic lentis
- Hypoplastic ciliary muscle
- Hypoplastic iris
- Increased axial length of the globe
- Myopia

Pulmonary System
- Apical blebs
- Spontaneous pneumothorax

M

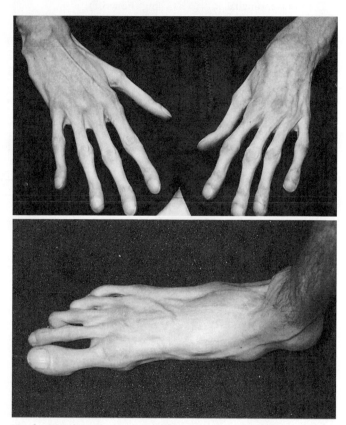

Marfan Syndrome. This young man has prominent arachnodactyly of both fingers and toes. Note the clubbing due to associated cardiopulmonary problems and the flattening of the arch of his foot. (*From Zitelli BJ, Davis HW:* Atlas of Pediatric Physical Diagnosis, *ed. 5, Philadelphia, 2007, Mosby.*)

Skeletal System

- Arachnodactyly
- Dolichocephaly
- Dolichostenomelia
- Downsloping palpebral fissures
- Enophthalmos
- High-arched palate with dental crowding
- Increased arm span–to-height ratio (>1.05)
- Joint hypermobility
- Malar hypoplasia
- Pectus carinatum
- Pectus excavatum
- Positive Steinberg sign (thumb extends beyond ulnar border when flexed in the palm)
- Positive wrist sign (thumb-index overlap when encircling the wrist)
- Progressive hindfoot collapse leading to pes planovalgus
- Protrusio acetabuli
- Reduced upper-to-lower segment ratio (distance from head to pubic symphysis divided by distance from pubic symphysis to soles) <0.85
- Retrognathia
- Scoliosis >20 degrees
- Spondylolisthesis
- Thoracolumbar scoliosis

Skin and Integumentary System

- Recurrent or incisional hernia
- Striae atrophicae not associated with pregnancy or repetitive stress

Medical Management

The primary focus of Marfan syndrome is the prevention of cardiovascular compromise. β-Blocking medications reduce inotrophy and chronotrophy as well as reduce the stress on the aorta, particularly the aortic root. Nitroprusside is added to the treatment regimen to lower the systemic vascular resistance, which reduces the afterload and reduces the stress on the heart. Combined administration of β blockers and nitroprusside provide a synergistic effect of reduced aortic stiffness, lower vascular resistance, and improved cardiac compliance.

Mitral valve prolapse frequently becomes so severe that surgical replacement is required. Often the defective valve is found to have a dilated annulus, redundant and flaccid cusps, and ruptured chordae tendineae. Frequently the ascending aorta and/or incompetent aortic valve must also be surgically repaired or replaced. Composite graft repair is the intervention of choice for a widely dilated ascending aorta, significantly attenuated aortic cusps, and acutely dissected aortic root. Composite grafting repair is also frequently recommended as a prophylactic measure for a patient with a history of increasing aortic dilation and/or a family history of sudden cardiovascular death.

Scoliosis is another symptom in Marfan syndrome for which surgical intervention is required. Nonsurgical management (conservative treatment) is often attempted initially, usually in the form of bracing, but it is not typically successful. Scoliosis curve progression in a Marfan syndrome patient may be as rapid as 7 to 10 degrees every year after onset of the disease. The degree of scoliosis combined with poor musculature and chest deformities can result in significant respiratory compromise. Chest wall deformities (specifically pectus excavatum) can be very severe—so severe, in fact, that cardiopulmonary function may be impaired. In such cases, the deformity can be surgically corrected to allow improvement of cardiopulmonary function.

Complications

- Abdominal aortic dilation
- Abdominal aortic dissection
- Aortic root dilation
- Aortic root dissection
- Bacterial endocarditis
- Cor pulmonale
- Death
- Descending aortic dilation
- Descending aortic dissection
- Heart failure
- Kyphotic deformity
- Mitral valve annulus calcification
- Mitral valve regurgitation
- Moderate-to-severe scoliosis
- Pneumothorax

Anesthesia Implications

The primary focus of the preoperative evaluation of a patient with Marfan syndrome concerns the cardiovascular system. Specifically, the focus is to determine the presence of imminent compromise or to specifically rule out imminent compromise. The cardiac evaluation must be thorough and include both electrocardiography and echocardiography. Aortic dilation, dissection, and rupture can develop quickly at any age. The anesthetist should guard against extreme fluctuations in blood pressure and, in particular, sustained elevation in blood pressure, as well as avoid sudden elevations in myocardial contractility because of the fragility of the patient's aorta. Administration of a β-blocking medication is useful in managing the patient's blood pressure.

The patient with Marfan syndrome is prone to valvular heart disease. Prophylactic antibiotic coverage is needed for any procedure that may put the patient at risk for development of bacteremia. This is especially true with regard to any dental procedures or surgical interventions.

The patient should be monitored invasively throughout the perioperative period, especially during longer, more intricate surgical procedures. The monitoring devices should include an arterial pressure catheter and a transesophageal echocardiograph, where available.

A patient with Marfan syndrome has loose joint ligaments and is prone to frequent joint dislocations. Of particular interest to the anesthetist is the frequency and relative ease with which the temporomandibular joint may dislocate. Joint laxity also affects the cervical spine. The patient must be carefully positioned to avoid injury to the cervical spine, including joint dislocations and subluxations. As a result, the anesthetist should anticipate that the patient will be difficult to intubate.

As mentioned above, hypertension in the patient with Marfan syndrome is particularly dangerous. Additionally, lability of blood pressure can be very detrimental. The periods of intubation and emergence/extubation are extremely stimulating events that are liable to compound the sympathetic stimulation. Adequate pain control is an integral aspect in controlling the blood pressure throughout the course of the anesthesia, from induction through the immediate postoperative period. In addition to pain control, anxiolysis is an important component and will work synergistically with pain control and β-blocking medications to better control the patient's blood pressure.

Mastocytosis

Definition

Mastocytosis is a clonal disorder in which mast cells and the precursor cells accumulate in different tissues, such as bone marrow, skin, gastrointestinal tract, liver, and spleen.

Classifications of Mastocytosis	
Category IA	Indolent disease with skin involvement
Category IB	Systemic involvement with or without skin involvement
Category II	A hematopoietic disorder is a part of the disease
Category IIA	Dysmyelopoietic disorder associated with mastocytosis
Category IIB	Accompanied by myeloproliferative disease
Category IIC	Associated with nonlymphocytic leukemia
Category IID	Associated with malignant lymphoma
Category IIE	Associated with neutropenia
Category III	Mast cell leukemia becomes a part of the disease
Category IV	Associated with lymphadenopathic mastocytosis with eosinophilia (also known as aggressive mastocytosis)

Incidence

The incidence of mastocytosis is extremely rare. The specific frequency of occurrence has not been documented.

Etiology

Mutations of the c-*kit* proto-oncogene have been implicated as the cause of some forms of mastocytosis. The systemic form, a codon-816 c-*kit* mutation, is commonly found.

Signs and Symptoms

- Abdominal pain
- Anemia
- Ascites
- Basophilia
- Budd-Chiari syndrome (see p. 59)
- Dilated small bowel
- Diverticulitis
- Eosinophilia
- Esophageal stricture
- Esophageal varices
- Esophagitis

M

- Hepatomegaly
- Leukocytosis
- Leukopenia
- Lymphadenopathy
- Lymphopenia
- Malabsorption
- Monocytosis
- Mucosal lesions
- Multiple polyposis
- Peptic ulcer disease
- Portal hypertension
- Sclerosing cholangitis
- Splenomegaly
- Thrombocytopenia
- Thrombocytosis

Medical Management

Medical interventions for the patient with mastocytosis are aimed mostly at symptomatic relief and are not curative. The primary goal is to institute measures directed toward decreasing the activation of mast cells. Mast cells are instrumental/integral participants in the allergic response. Mast cell activation causes release of substances stored within the cell (i.e., histamine, heparin, prostaglandin D_2), resulting in signs and symptoms of a severe allergic response, even anaphylaxis. Epinephrine is the treatment of choice for the appearance of a severe allergic or anaphylactic reaction. H_1- and H_2-blocking medications may also be useful in controlling anaphylactic symptoms.

Peptic ulcer disease associated with mastocytosis may be treated by administration of H_2-blocking medications to reduce the gastric hypersecretion. Proton pump inhibitors are also an effective treatment in peptic ulcer disease.

Pruritus is often treated with psoralen ultraviolet A, which has been reported to provide transient relief, but it may also cause some patients' skin lesions to fade. Diarrhea associated with mastocytosis may be treated with administration of either anticholinergics or disodium cromolyn. Various chemotherapeutic medications are used to treat Categories II to IV of systemic mastocytosis. The results have not yet been successful. The two medications most often used are interferon alfa and 2-chlorodeoxyadenosine.

Allogenic bone marrow transplantation is being studied in clinical trials by the National Institutes of Health to treat the bone marrow infiltration, but this intervention is considered experimental.

Diagnostic surgical interventions such as laparoscopy, bone marrow biopsy, and endoscopy may exacerbate the condition. These interventions may activate the mast cells and precipitate an anaphylactic response.

Hematologic Manifestations Associated with Mastocytosis

- Castleman disease
- Hairy-cell leukemia
- Hypereosinophilic syndrome
- Monoclonal gammopathy
- Non-Hodgkin's lymphoma
- Polycythemia vera
- Primary thrombocytopenia

Complications

- Anaphylaxis
- Death
- Hepatomegaly
- Lymphadenopathy
- Malabsorption
- Pathologic fractures
- Prolonged clotting times
- Splenomegaly

Anesthesia Implications

Preoperative laboratory data should be extensive and include liver enzymes, complete blood count, metabolic panel as well as prothrombin, partial thromboplastin, and bleeding times. Liver involvement can alter or delay the metabolism and elimination of most anesthesia-related medications. Derangements in PT/PTT and bleeding times, along with low platelet counts, must be addressed before initiating the proposed surgery. Treatments include platelet transfusion(s), vitamin K administration, and infusion of fresh frozen plasma.

The patient's fluid and electrolyte status should be assessed before initiating any form of surgery and anesthesia. These parameters are particularly important for the patient with significant involvement of the gastrointestinal system. Proliferation of mast cells in the GI tract can result in a malabsorption syndrome. The malabsorption affects both fluid and electrolyte concentrations. In addition, malabsorption interferes with appropriate protein synthesis, which can have far-reaching effects on the actions of many anesthesia-related drugs and alter the production of clotting factors. Inadequate serum proteins result in greater bioavailability of protein-bound medications. Low serum proteins also contribute to loss of free water intravascularly, leading to dehydration.

Bony infiltration is also a prominent characteristic of mastocytosis. The lesions, which are very painful, may be osteoporotic or osteosclerotic. Bone pain indicates a higher potential for pathologic fractures. A great concern for the anesthetist is the positioning of the patient. Exaggerated gentleness is necessary to minimize the potential for fractures during the perioperative period.

The anesthetist must strive to avoid mast cell activation, which results in histamine release. Histamine release may occur as the result of physical, psychological, or chemical stimulation. Anxiolysis is important for the patient with mastocytosis. Adding an antihistamine to the premedication regimen may be beneficial. The anesthetist must also strictly avoid medications closely associated with the release of histamine, such as morphine, codeine, atropine, dextran, and sodium thiopental. Physical stimulation can also trigger histamine release. Therefore the anesthetist and OR staff should absolutely minimize rubbing the patient's skin. In addition, the patient should not be allowed to experience extremes in ambient temperature, which will lead to shivering—a very potent physical stimulant. The patient must be kept warm throughout the surgical procedure, and any fluids should be warmed before they are administered.

The patient with mastocytosis is prone to anaphylactic reactions. As such, the anesthetist must be prepared at any instant to treat an anaphylactic reaction, or any sudden, unexplained episode of hypotension during the perioperative period. The anesthetist must have appropriate medications immediately at hand before induction of anesthesia, including epinephrine and other catecholamines, antihistamines, and/or bronchodilators.

M

Myasthenia Gravis

Definition

Myasthenia gravis is an acquired autoimmune disorder of neuromuscular function marked by fatigue and exhaustion of the muscular system. Fluctuations in severity of muscular atrophy accompany periods of increased or decreased activity.

Incidence

Myasthenia gravis is not very common. It is estimated to occur at a rate of 2:1,000,000.

Etiology

Myasthenia gravis is caused by the presence of antibodies against acetylcholine receptors at the neuromuscular junction of skeletal muscles; 80% to 90% of myasthenia gravis patients have antibodies against acetylcholine receptors. Tolerance to acetylcholine receptors by the immune system is somehow lost, but the mechanism is not clear. Myasthenia gravis is considered to be a B-cell–mediated disease process; however, T-cells' contribution to the process is becoming increasingly more evident. T-cell immunity is dominated by the thymus, and myasthenia gravis patients frequently have thymic hyperplasia, thymoma, or other thymus abnormalities.

Signs and Symptoms

- Acute respiratory failure
- Aspiration
- Difficulty chewing
- Difficulty swallowing
- Horizontal smile
- Hyperthyroidism
- Lupus
- Mask-like facies
- Nasal regurgitation of food and liquids
- Ophthalmoplegia
- Proptosis (exophthalmos)
- Ptosis
- Rheumatoid arthritis
- Scleroderma

M

Myasthenia Gravis Foundation of America Clinical Classifications

Class I
- Any ocular muscle weakness
- May have weakness of eye closure
- All other muscle strength is normal

Class II
- Mild weakness affecting other than ocular muscles
- May have ocular muscle weakness of any severity

Class IIa
- Predominately affecting limb or axial muscles or both
- May also have lesser involvement of oropharyngeal muscles

Class IIb
- Predominately affecting oropharyngeal or respiratory muscles or both
- May also have lesser or equal involvement of limb or axial muscles or both

Class III
- Moderate weakness affecting other than ocular muscles
- May also have ocular muscle weakness of any severity

Class IIIa
- Predominately affecting limb or axial muscles or both

- May also have lesser involvement of oropharyngeal muscles

Class IIIb
- Predominately affects oropharyngeal or respiratory muscles or both
- May also have lesser or equal involvement of limb or axial muscles or both

Class IV
- Predominately affects limb and/or axial muscles
- May also have lesser involvement of oropharyngeal muscles

Class IVb
- Predominantely affects oropharyngeal or respiratory muscles or both
- May also have lesser involvement of oropharyngeal muscles
- Use of a feeding tube without intubation

Class V
- Defined by intubation, with or without ventilation, except when used during routine postoperative management
- Use of a feeding tube with intubation

Medical Management

Currently no rigorous treatment trials have been reported and there is no consensus regarding treatment regimens. Initiation and/or alteration of treatment regimens must take into account disease severity, distribution of affected muscles, and rapidity of progression. Acetylcholinesterase inhibitors and immunomodulation are stalwarts in treating myasthenia gravis. Plasmapheresis and thymectomy are nontraditional immunomodulation therapies that have been employed.

Plasma exchange is an effective therapy before surgery or as an effective short-term management response to an acute exacerbation of the disease. The improvement in strength is helpful in reducing postoperative recovery time and may contribute to reduction of the length of ventilatory assistance. Muscle weakness is improved days after treatment initiation, but the improvement lasts only 6 to 8 weeks. Plasma exchange can be used as a long-term treatment for the patient who has not responded to other treatment regimens. The primary limitation of plasma exchange has been the difficulty of gaining intravenous access, but hypotension and coagulation derangements are also possible. Central venous access should be obtained for the patient receiving plasma exchange treatments.

Surgical intervention in the form of thymectomy is a very important option for myasthenia gravis patients. Some experts advocate this option as the first-line therapeutic intervention, particularly for patients with generalized myasthenia gravis and those with thymoma. Despite the absence of controlled trials to investigate the efficacy of thymectomy, this intervention has become the *de facto* standard of care for patients with thymoma or for those from 10 to 55 years of age with generalized myasthenia gravis. Disease remission may result from thymectomy, typically in younger patients who have been affected for only a short time, those with hyperplastic thymus, and those with high antibody titers. The frequency of remission increases over time; 7 to 10 years post-surgery, 40% to 60% of all thymectomy patients experience remission.

Drugs that Can Exacerbate Myasthenia Gravis Symptoms

- Antibiotics (aminoglycosides, ciprofloxacin, erythromycin, ampicillin)
- Anticholinergics (such as trihexyphenidyl)
- β-adrenergic blocking agents (propranolol, oxprenolol)
- Chloroquine
- Lithium
- Magnesium
- Prednisone
- Procainamide
- Quinidine
- Timolol (Blocadren)
- Verapamil

Complications

- Aspiration pneumonia
- Avascular necrosis
- Cataracts
- Dysphagia
- Fungal infections (systemic)
- Gastritis
- Hyperglycemia
- Lymphoproliferative
  malignancies

- Osteoporosis
- Peptic ulcer disease
- *Pneumocystis jiroveci*
  pneumonia
- Respiratory failure
- Teratogenic fetal effects
- Tuberculosis
- Weight gain

Anesthesia Implications

Immunomodulation requires renewed attention to antisepsis from the anesthetist. As a result of immunomodulation therapy, the patient may be more susceptible to opportunistic infection(s) and the anesthetist is involved in potentially hazardous aspects of antigen introduction: intravenous access and endotracheal intubation.

As part of immunomodulation therapy, corticosteroids are frequently incorporated into the treatment regimen. If steroids are a part of the patient's treatment regimen, a perioperative stress dose of steroid will be needed.

Muscular weakness is a critical factor for the anesthetist to consider. The patient with myasthenia gravis is exquisitely sensitive to nondepolarizing muscle relaxants. For surgical procedures that require relaxation, the smallest effective dose should be administered. Minimizing the dose will increase the potential effectiveness of reversal medication if it is needed. The anesthetist is cautioned that ulnar nerve stimulation may demonstrate deceptively greater muscle strength than the patient actually has, and additional criteria should be employed for assessing the return of adequate muscle strength to allow for extubation. Even with these alterations, the anesthetist and the patient must recognize the very real possibility of prolonged effects from the muscle relaxants and all parties (patient, family, anesthetist, and surgeon) should be prepared for the potential need for postoperative ventilatory support. Postoperative ventilatory support is often continued via tracheal intubation with mechanical ventilation for a period of time to allow the patient to "naturally" regain the requisite muscle strength. However, even after regaining sufficient muscle strength for extubation, the patient with myasthenia gravis may succumb to fatigue and require re-intubation.

Intubation, at any time, of the patient with myasthenia gravis does not necessarily require administration of muscle relaxants. In addition to being extremely sensitive to nondepolarizing relaxants, the patient is resistant to the depolarizing muscle relaxants, such as succinylcholine. The response to a dose of succinylcholine is unpredictable. The patient with myasthenia gravis is prone to develop a Phase II block, even at the reduced succinylcholine dose of 0.5 mg/kg, and recovery from the Phase II block is a slow process. In contrast, it may be difficult to pharmacologically produce muscle relaxation because of the patient's anticholinesterase therapy. Chronic anticholinesterase therapy also produces other effects, such as potentiation of vagal responses, reduced metabolism of ester-type local anesthetics, and increased duration and efficacy of narcotics. Because ester-type local anesthetics are not easily metabolized by patients with myasthenia gravis, this class of local agents may be more toxic for them than amide-type local anesthetics. Postoperative resumption of anticholinesterase therapy must be based on the outcome of the edrophonium test. Dosage requirements for anticholinesterase medications change, particularly during the postoperative period.

M

Narcolepsy

Definition

A neurologic disorder, narcolepsy is a derangement of the
normal sleep-wake cycle characterized by episodes of excessive daytime sleepiness (EDS), cataplexy, hypnagogic and/or
hypnopompic hallucinations, and sleep paralysis, all of which
represent inappropriate intrusions of sleep into the awake state.
Onset of this disorder may be at any time, from as young as
10 years of age through the fifth decade. There is no known
cure at the present time.

Incidence

Narcolepsy is found worldwide without regard to race or ethnic
group. Some groups appear to be more prone to develop narcolepsy; in Japan the estimated incidence is 1:600, in the United
States the estimated prevalence ranges from 1:1000 to 1:10,000,
and in Israel the estimated prevalence is 1:500,000. The estimated
prevalence rates for the United States, alone, may account for
10,000 to 20,000 to as many as 100,000 to 200,000 patients.

Etiology

The cause of narcolepsy has not been delineated. The disease
does seem to appear in families.

Signs and Symptoms

The classic symptoms of narcolepsy include EDS, cataplexy, sleep
paralysis, and hypnogogic or hypnopompic hallucinations, which
are referred to as the "narcolepsy tetrad." When a patient reports
EDS that is accompanied by one of the other three parts of the
tetrad, the diagnosis of narcolepsy is highly suspected. Only 20% to
25% of patients with narcolepsy display all four parts of the tetrad.

Medical Management

Narcolepsy is incurable. Occasionally, some patients are able
to treat EDS by scheduling nap periods over the course of the

day. More frequently, patients with narcolepsy must depend on pharmacologic support to treat symptoms. EDS/sleep attacks are treated using central nervous system stimulants. Cataplexy may be treated with tricyclic antidepressants (TCAs)or possibly fluoxetine.

Complications

Complications that may arise do so from increased risk of injury resulting from excessive daytime sleepiness or cataplexy.

Anesthetic Implications

The major anesthetic implications of narcolepsy revolve around medication interactions. Enzyme induction with a patient who has narcolepsy can be expected secondary to treatment with CNS stimulants and/or tricyclic antidepressants. The CNS stimulants and tricyclic antidepressants used for symptomatic treatment are metabolized by the liver.

Most of the CNS stimulants employed are noncatechol-amine sympathomimetic amines. Long-term administration of amphetamines may reduce the anesthetic requirements.

Response to ephedrine or phenylephrine may be exaggerated. Response to atropine may be exaggerated in patients taking tricyclic antidepressants.

Sedation from sodium thiopental is prolonged in the patient taking a TCA. Acute hypertension and cardiac dysrhythmias may occur with the administration of ketamine.

Cataplexy, a state of paralysis in which the patient is fully conscious but unable to move, is triggered by extremes in emotion, excitement, stress, surprise, or startle. All these factors may be experienced in a patient emerging from anesthesia. Other potential causes of immobility must be investigated before concentrating on the possibility of an episode of cataplexy being the cause of immobility. In the event that cataplexy is the cause, support and calm reassurance are the most appropriate measures to take. The anesthetist should communicate understanding of the situation at hand and may administer a small dose of an IV sedative to alleviate any anxiety the patient may be experiencing.

Hypnopompic hallucinations may occur during emergence from general anesthesia or any situation in which the patient has received heavy sedation. This patient may act out or act on the event he or she perceives. The patient may be inordinately frightened and/or combative during the emergence process. Calm yet firm reassurance combined with small increments of IV sedation will help the patient through such an episode.

Sleep paralysis may occur during emergence from general anesthesia, during a regional anesthetic, or during a monitored care case. This symptom is very similar to cataplexy but may be distinguished from cataplexy by the patient's ability to open his or her eyes spontaneously. As with the other symptoms of the narcolepsy tetrad, calm reassurance and possibly a small amount of IV sedation may be the best course of action to aid and comfort the patient.

N

> ## Nephrotic Syndrome

Definition

Nephrotic syndrome is a clinical condition or group of disorders that involves defective kidney glomeruli with massive proteinuria, lipiduria with edema, hypoalbuminemia, and hyperlipidemia. It is classified as either primary nephrotic syndrome (PNS), formerly termed idiopathic nephrotic syndrome, or secondary nephrotic syndrome.

Incidence

The incidence of nephrotic syndrome for patients younger than 16 years of age is 2:100,000 to 5:100,000. For the total population, the incidence is 15.5:100,000.

Etiology

For nephrotic syndrome, a glomerular cause is generally accepted. The specific initiating event or root cause producing the massive proteinuria is still undetermined, although an immune pathology is strongly suspected. The permeability of the glomerular basement membrane is altered and the capillary transport of albumin, an anionically charged molecule, is increased by a deficiency of sialic acid from the basement membrane.

Signs and Symptoms

- Abdominal discomfort
- Albuminuria
- Anasarca
- Anorexia
- Ascites
- Azotemia
- Diarrhea
- Fatigue
- Fever
- Hematuria
- Hyperlipidemia
- Hypoalbuminemia
- Hypoproteinemia
- Hypotension
- Irritability
- Lipiduria
- Massive proteinuria
- Pallor
- Pitting edema
- Tachypnea

N

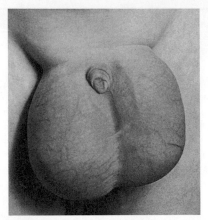

Nephrotic Syndrome. Severe scrotal edema in a 6-year-old with nephrotic syndrome. *(From Zitelli BJ, Davis HW:* Atlas of Pediatric Physical Diagnosis, *ed. 5, St. Louis, 2007, Mosby.)*

Medical Management

The agent of choice to treat nephrotic syndrome is a gluco-corticoid, typically prednisone or prednisolone. High-dose therapy is employed if no contraindications to that therapy are present. The initial regimen is continued for 4 to 8 weeks. Maintenance with prednisone or prednisolone is recommended for the next 6 months on an alternating-day schedule and is tapered downward to discontinuation over the course of those 6 months.

Patients with nephrotic syndrome are at higher risk for opportunistic infection. Treatment with the glucocorticoid(s) produces immune system modulation and contributes sig-nificantly to this increased vulnerability. Any time the patient with nephrotic syndrome is febrile or demonstrates signs and symptoms of infection, close observation is warranted until the infectious organism is determined. Once the organism is identified, aggressive treatment must be initiated.

Pitting edema is treated, especially when it is symptomatic. Loop diuretics are effective but must be administered with cau-tion. Diuresis can exacerbate plasma volume concentration that may already be present, resulting in intense hypovolemia and possibly hypovolemic shock. If the edema is of such magnitude

N

to require diuretic therapy, an infusion of salt-poor albumin should be administered simultaneously.

Hypertension should be treated when it is demonstrated, especially if it is persistent. Occasionally, hypertension responds to diuretic therapy. The preferred treatment consists of administration of an angiotensin-converting enzyme inhibitor (ACEI) or with an angiotensin II–receptor antagonist (A2RA). Short-term treatment may be effectively accomplished using a calcium channel–blocking medication; however, hypertension with significantly persistent proteinuria is best treated with either an ACEI or an A2RA.

An integral part of the treatment regimen for the patient with nephrotic syndrome is teaching the patient to monitor urinary protein/albumin at home. The easiest, simplest, and least expensive method is generally sufficient. Urine dipsticks are typically used, but turbidity tests such as sulfosalicylic acid may be used. The patient is strongly encouraged to initiate and maintain a journal recording the results of each at-home test, which is usually done every morning. This follow-up method is particularly important once the patient's urine has become protein free. Detection of urinary protein may signify recurrence of the disease well before the development of edema and allows for initiation of treatment measures much sooner.

Complications

- Acute renal failure
- Cataracts
- Chronic renal failure
- End-stage renal disease
- Glomerular lesion
- Growth arrest
- Hirsutism
- Hyperglycemia
- Hyperlipidemia
- Hypoproteinemia
- Mild psychoses
- Moonface
- Nephrolithiasis
- Obesity
- Osteopenia
- Osteoporosis
- Persistent hypertension
- Thromboembolism
- Toxic effects of individual drugs (i.e., antihypertensives, immunosuppressants, cyclophosphamide, chlorambucil, cyclosporine)
- Tubulointerstitial nephritis

Anesthesia Implications

The anesthetist must be mindful of aseptic technique when interacting with the patient with nephrotic syndrome. The patient is immunomodulated by virtue of the administration of glucocorticosteroids for treatment of the syndrome, and so is at higher risk for opportunistic infection. The "simple" acts of obtaining intravenous access and endotracheal intubation should be accomplished using strict aseptic technique. Prophylactic antibiotic coverage with a broad-spectrum agent may be prudent.

The patient's fluid and electrolyte status should be assessed preoperatively. Attention should be paid to the concentration of serum proteins as well. Hypoproteinemia can significantly alter the bioavailability of highly protein-bound drugs, such as midazolam or sodium thiopental. If serum proteins are low at the time of induction, the doses of such drugs should be reduced.

The patient's renal function should be evaluated preoperatively. For the patient with nephrotic syndrome, greater reliance should be placed on the serum indicators, such as blood urea nitrogen and serum creatinine. The anesthetist is cautioned to be somewhat skeptical about urine output, particularly if the patient is receiving diuretic therapy.

The patient may still be receiving the maintenance dose of glucocorticosteroids or may have recently discontinued steroid therapy. In either event, a stress dose of a steroid is an appropriate measure.

N

Neurofibromatosis

Definition

Neurofibromatosis is a familial, multisystem, genetic disorder characterized by developmental changes in the nervous system, muscles, bones, and skin. It is marked by the formation of neurofibromas over the entire body and associated with areas of pigmentation. Neurofibromatosis is also known as von Recklinghausen's disease.

Incidence

The estimated frequency of neurofibromatosis is 1:3000 to 1:4000 people. The actual incidence may be higher.

Etiology

The cause of neurofibromatosis is mutation or deletion of the *NF1* gene, which is found on the long arm of chromosome 17, resulting in decreased production of neurofibromin. The precise role of neurofibromin is still not fully understood, but this gene product has a multitude of effects and diverse functions in several tissues.

Diagnostic Criteria for Neurofibromatosis

Diagnosis requires the presence of two or more of the following seven criteria:

1. Six or more café-au-lait spots or hyperpigmented macules (5 mm in diameter for children younger than 10 years of age or 15 mm in adults)
2. Axillary or inguinal freckles
3. Two or more neurofibromas or one plexiform neurofibroma
4. Two or more iris hamartomas (Lisch nodules)
5. Sphenoid dysplasia or long-bone abnormalities (e.g., pseudoarthrosis)
6. First-degree relative with neurofibromatosis
7. Optic nerve glioma

N

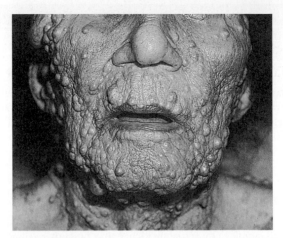

Neurofibromatosis. Neurofibromas. *(From Swartz MH:* Textbook of Physical Diagnosis: History and Examination, *ed. 5, Philadelphia, 2006, Saunders.)*

Signs and Symptoms

- Axillary or inguinal freckles
- Café-au-lait spots
- Congenital pseudoarthrosis
- Forearm bowing
- Hypertension
- Macrocephaly
- Noncorrectable vision loss
- Optic nerve tumors
- Plexiform neurofibromas with or without hypertrichosis or hyperpigmentation
- Pruritus
- Scoliosis with or without kyphosis
- Sphenoid bone dysplasia
- Subcutaneous or cutaneous neurofibromas
- Thinning and angulation of long bones

Medical Management

Physical examination(s) should be performed at least annually and should focus on detection of potential complications. Early detection helps reduce morbidity and improves the patient's quality of life. Each annual examination should look for development of new neurofibromas and document the progression of previously existing fibromas.

N

Physical Examination Documentation for the Patient with Neurofibromatosis

- *Blood pressure:* Evaluate on every visit; treat hypertension promptly; evaluate for pheochromocytoma or renal artery stenosis
- *Cutaneous examination:* Neurofibromas or progression of existing neurofibromas; evidence of bony erosion or nerve entrapment
- *Neurologic:* Development of paresthesia or radiculopathy; weakness or muscle atrophy; incontinence; symptoms of spinal cord neurofibromas
- *Skeletal:* Scoliosis, hemihypertrophy, long-bone modeling defects

Surgical Interventions for the Patient with Neurofibromatosis

- Angioplasty for renal artery stenosis
- Peripheral nerve sheath tumors, particularly along the brachial and/or sacral plexuses
- Pseudoarthrosis; may require amputation despite attempts at bracing, casting, or other limb-sparing interventions
- Resection and grafting of renal artery stenosis
- Resection for neurofibromas pressing on vital structures, obstructing vision, or growing rapidly
- Resection of neurofibromas for cosmetic and/or aesthetic reasons
- Spinal cord tumor excision

Aside from periodic examination and evaluation, there is no medical therapy that is documented or known to be beneficial to patients with neurofibromatosis. At times pruritus associated with cutaneous neurofibromas may respond to the administration of diphenhydramine; also, carboplatin combined with vincristine sulfate has demonstrated efficacy in treating optic nerve lesions. Surgical interventions include resection of neurofibromas that create cosmetic/aesthetic concerns or that encroach or press on vital structures, obstruct vision, or grow rapidly.

Complications

- Attention deficit disorder
- Attention deficit hyperactivity disorder
- Brachial plexus neurofibroma
- Brain tumors
- Cervical kyphosis
- Dumbbell-shaped spinal cord neurofibromas
- Hypertension secondary to pheochromocytoma
- Kyphosis
- Learning disabilities
- Leukemia
- Locally invasive plexiform neurofibromas
- Long-bone congenital bowing
- Mental retardation
- Neural crest origin malignancies
- Optic nerve lesions
- Paraplegia
- Pathologic fractures
- Peripheral neuropathy
- Pseudoarthrosis
- Renal vascular stenosis secondary to fibromuscular dysplasia
- Sacral plexus neurofibroma
- Sacrolumbar meningocele
- Scoliosis
- Thoracic cage asymmetry
- Tibial pseudoarthrosis

Anesthesia Implications

Because neurofibromas may originate virtually anywhere in the patient's body, the airway must be thoroughly—almost exhaustively—evaluated. The evaluation should include computed tomography (CT), magnetic resonance imaging (MRI), and/or indirect laryngoscopy. Use of a laryngeal mask airway may be appropriate for many surgical procedures. Neurofibromas may obstruct the patient's airway on induction of general anesthesia. The patient may quickly become a "can't ventilate/can't intubate" patient. It may be necessary to secure the airway via awake fiberoptic means. Fiberoptic methods may not be successful and a tracheotomy may be required to secure the patient's airway.

Pulmonary complaints and exercise tolerance should be carefully documented. A patient with kyphoscoliosis and chronic lung disease should be evaluated with chest x-ray, arterial blood gas analysis, static and dynamic lung volume determinations, and forced expiratory volumes (gas flow rates).

N

Regional anesthesia is an entirely appropriate technique for the patient with neurofibromatosis. However, the patient's back should be closely examined when considering whether to use regional anesthesia for the proposed surgical procedure. The anesthetist must remember that asymptomatic interspace neurofibromas, sacrolumbar meningocele, or severe kyphoscoliosis may seriously impede or completely obstruct identification of and/or entry into the epidural or subarachnoid space.

Pathologic fractures are one of the many complications associated with neurofibromatosis. The anesthetist must take great caution in positioning the patient and ensuring that adequate and proper padding of extremities and other pressure points is provided.

The patient should be evaluated for the presence of a pheochromocytoma by determining the urinary catecholamine concentrations. The anesthetist must have medications to treat a hypertensive crisis easily within reach to avoid any treatment delay.

As yet, no anesthetic drug or technique is strongly recommended for the patient with neurofibromatosis. If the patient has spinal cord lesions higher than the midthoracic level, the condition may be complicated by the development of autonomic hyperreflexia and all its myriad implications. The patient with significant muscle atrophy or wasting should probably not receive succinylcholine.

N

Neuroleptic Malignant Syndrome

Definition

Neuroleptic malignant syndrome (NMS) is a potentially fatal, iatrogenic syndrome characterized by hyperpyrexia, catatonic rigidity, mentation alteration, and profuse sweating. Rhabdomyolysis, renal failure, seizures, and death have also been reported in association with NMS.

Incidence

Reportedly 0.02% to 3.25% of all patients to whom antipsychotic, neuroleptic, or dopamine-antagonizing medications are administered develop NMS. The box lists risk factors associated with the development of NMS.

Risk Factors for Neuroleptic Malignant Syndrome

- Age (young to middle-aged adult)
- Antipsychotic medication ingestion
- D_2 dopamine-antagonist ingestion
- Dehydration
- Exhaustion
- Male sex
- Neuroleptic medication ingestion
- Psychiatric illness
- Psychomotor activity/agitation

Etiology

Current evidence seems to indicate that an acute reduction in dopamine activity in the brain is the basic mechanism for the development of NMS. Dopamine-antagonist medications have been implicated in the development of NMS. The risk of developing NMS is related to dosage, potency, and rate and route of administration.

An NMS episode may be preceded by a number of rather nonspecific "prodromal" signs (see box on facing page). The onset of an episode typically occurs within 7 to 10 days after the intake of any of the implicated associated medications. Development of an episode of NMS does not indicate an overdose of a medication; rather, NMS seems to develop in reaction to dosages within the therapeutic range. Onset of an episode of NMS mimics the onset of malignant hyperthermia (MH).

N

There are other pathologies that must be considered in the differential process, including local or systemic infection, seizure disorder, thyroid storm, pheochromocytoma, central nervous system tumor, or cerebrovascular accident, as well as ingestion or overdose of a medication or sudden discontinuation of a medication. The box below provides diagnostic criteria for NMS.

Prodromal Signs of Neuroleptic Malignant Syndrome

- Catatonia
- Diaphoresis
- Dysarthria
- Dysphagia
- Hypertension
- Low-grade fever of unknown origin
- Myoclonus
- Obtundation
- Sialorrhea
- Sudden mentation alteration
- Tachycardia
- Tachypnea
- Tremor

Diagnostic Criteria for Neuroleptic Malignant Syndrome

*Simultaneous occurrence of five of the following, **plus** numbers 1 to 4 below:*

- Diaphoresis or sialorrhea
- Hypertension/hypotension
- Incontinence
- Increased creatinine phosphokinase
- Leukocytosis
- Mental status change
- Metabolic acidosis
- Myoglobinuria
- Tachycardia
- Tremor

1. Neuroleptic treatment within the previous 2 to 4 weeks
2. Hyperthermia
3. Muscle rigidity
4. Drug-induced systemic or neuropsychiatric illnesses have been ruled out

Signs and Symptoms

- Altered mental status
- Diaphoresis
- Elevated creatinine phosphokinase
- Elevated urinary myoglobin
- Hypertension or hypotension
- Hyperthermia (>100.4° F [>38° C])
- Incontinence
- Leukocytosis
- Metabolic acidosis
- Muscle rigidity
- Sialorrhea
- Tachycardia
- Tachypnea
- Tremor

N

Medical Management

Early recognition of NMS is critical. As with any negative effect of a medication, immediate discontinuation is required when it is recognized. This is critical because NMS may not manifest itself for 24 hours to 30 days *after* exposure to a triggering medication. It may well be the case that the decision to discontinue medication was made before the anesthetist became involved in the patient's treatment. The actions typically initiated by the anesthetist are intense, supportive/palliative measures focusing at first primarily on fluid administration, hydration maintenance, temperature reduction, and cardiac/pulmonary/renal function support as dictated by the developing, ongoing situation. Until definitive diagnosis is obtained, initiation of the facility's malignant hyperthermia (MH) protocol is warranted (see box below). Because the patient may become agitated as a result of NMS, benzodiazepine administration may be warranted. Nondepolarizing muscle relaxants (NDMRs) may be instrumental in halting the muscle rigidity the patient may experience and may be an aid to a definitive diagnosis of NMS as opposed to MH; NDMRs will relax the patient with NMS but have no effect on the MH patient.

Treatment of Neuroleptic Malignant Syndrome

Immediate Treatment

Initiate the facility's Malignant Hyperthermia protocol as quickly as possible, including removal of all traces of anesthetic agents, exchange of anesthesia machine if feasible, hyperventilation with 100% oxygen, and cool packs to the axillae and groin.

Initiate administration of dantrolene at 1 to 2 mg/kg, with a maximum dose of 10 mg/kg/day, until diagnosis of NMS is confirmed. These measures will reduce thermogenesis and buy time.

Treatment after NMS Diagnosis Confirmed

Administer bromocriptine at 7.5 to 60 mg/day in divided doses. This drug can only be administered either by mouth or through a nasogastric tube. Symptomatic treatment following the Malignant Hyperthermia protocol should be provided to allow time for the onset of action by bromocriptine. Bromocriptine is a direct dopamine agonist, which will counteract the dopamine antagonists. Hypotension, delirium, and exacerbation of any underlying psychiatric disorder may accompany administration of bromocriptine.

N

Complications

- Acute renal failure
- Cardiac arrest
- Cardiac failure
- Disseminated intravascular coagulation (DIC)
- Ileus
- Myocardial infarction
- Myoglobinuric renal failure
- Pneumonia
- Pulmonary embolism
- Respiratory arrest
- Respiratory failure

Anesthesia Implications

Because the onset of NMS may occur 24 hours to 30 days after exposure to an implicated medication, the anesthetist may first encounter this disorder after induction of general anesthesia or administration of a regional anesthetic. NMS is so strikingly similar to MH that initial thought and treatment objectives must be directed as if MH is being experienced.

A thorough preoperative history is an essential component of care. The anesthetist should obtain a thorough pharmacologic history for the preceding 30 days, including prescription or over-the-counter self-medication, herbal medications, and illicit drug intake. Mortality for NMS is currently estimated at approximately 11%.

N

Osler-Weber-Rendu Syndrome

Definition

Osler-Weber-Rendu syndrome (OWRS) is an autosomal dominant, inherited disorder characterized by telangiectases, recurrent epistaxis, and first-degree relative(s) positive for the disorder. Telangiectases are lesions produced by telangiectasia. They may present as a coarse or fine, red line or may appear as a punctum with radiating arms (spider-like appearance). Osler-Weber-Rendu syndrome is also known as hereditary hemorrhagic telangiectasia (HHT).

Incidence

The incidence of OWRS is 1:100,000 to 2:100,000. It is reported in all racial groups and almost all ethnic groups without predilection for either gender.

Curaçao Criteria for Osler-Weber-Rendu Syndrome
• *Epistaxis:* Spontaneous and recurrent
• *Family history:* First-degree relative positive for hereditary hemorrhagic telangiectasia
• *Telangiectases:* Multiple at various characteristic sites (lips, oral cavity, fingers, nose)
• *Visceral lesions:* Gastrointestinal telangiectasia, pulmonary AVM, hepatic AVM, central AVM, or spinal AVM

AVM, Arteriovenous malformation.

Etiology

There are four types of HHT: (1) HHT type 1, (2) HHT type 2, (3) JPHT, and (4) HHT type 3. Genetic loci have been identified for three types of the disease. HHT type 1 results from defects in the long arm of chromosome 9 (9q33-34). HHT type 2 is derived from defects on the long arm of chromosome 12 (12q13). JPHT appears to result from mutations on the long arm of chromosome 5 (5q31.1-32). HHT type 3 appears to follow pathways similar to the three other types, but a specific gene locus has not been identified.

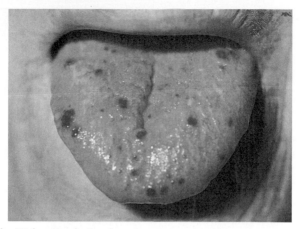

Osler-Weber-Rendu Syndrome. Note the telangiectatic lesions. *(From Swartz MH: Textbook of Physical Diagnosis: History and Examination, ed. 5, Philadelphia, 2006, Saunders.)*

Signs and Symptoms

- Anemia
- Arteriovenous malforma-
  tions (AVM) at multiple
  sites, notably the brain
  and lungs
- Clubbing
- Continuous thoracic bruit
- Cyanosis
- Dyspnea on exertion
- Easy fatigability
- Epistaxis
- Hemoptysis
- Hepatomegaly
- Jaundice
- Migraine
- Pallor
- Paraparesis
- Polycythemia
- Seizure
- Tachypnea
- Telangiectases of skin,
  mucous membranes, liver,
  brain, and spleen

Medical Management

Medical care for the patient with HHT focuses on decreasing hemorrhage, minimizing blood loss, and minimizing sequelae from chronic blood loss. The most common source of blood loss is recurrent epistaxis. The epistaxis may be treated via several methods, including humidification, nasal packing, estrogen therapy, aminocaproic acid, electrocautery, laser ablation, and

---

Hereditary Hemorrhagic Telangiectasia: Medical Interventions by Specific Affected Area

- *Central nervous system AVM.* Embolization/embolotherapy, stereotactic radiosurgery
- *Epistaxis:* Humidification, packing, estrogen therapy, aminocaproic acid, electrocautery, ND:YAG laser ablation, transfusion
- *GI bleeding:* Estrogen/progesterone therapy, aminocaproic acid, endoscopic photoablation, electrocautery, transfusion
- *Pulmonary AVM:* Embolization via transluminal deployment of a balloon or coil
- *Skin lesion:* Laser ablation, hypertonic saline sclerotherapy, topical medications

AVM, Arteriovenous malformation; *ND:YAG,* neodymium-yttrium-garnet.

septal dermoplasty. Blood transfusion may be necessary to correct chronic blood losses.

Surgical interventions may be indicated for several body areas. Epistaxis may be severe enough to warrant septal dermoplasty. Arteriovenous malformations (AVMs) are somewhat weakened outcroppings within the arterial-venous continuum and are prone to enlargement and rupture over time. AVMs are characteristic of OWRS and are particularly disconcerting when they are found in the lungs and/or brain, where rupture can lead to rapid demise. Surgical resection may be undertaken to avert/avoid rupture of an AVM and any potential associated untoward sequelae.

Gastrointestinal bleeding may occur episodically and may be a contributing source of chronic blood loss. Surgical intervention for gastrointestinal bleeding is indicated if the episode is believed to be a massive hemorrhagic event.

Complications

- Abdominal angina
- Brain abscess
- Encephalopathy
- Epidural hematoma
- Hemoptysis
- High-output heart failure
- Intraocular hemorrhage
- Ischemic stroke
- Mesenteric arterial "steal"
- Paradoxical emboli
- Paraparesis
- Portal hypertension
- Pseudocirrhosis
- Severe right-to-left pulmonary shunt
- Subarachnoid hemorrhage
- Transient ischemic attack

Anesthesia Implications

Telangiectatic lesions may occur throughout the body, including mucous membranes. While carrying out endotracheal
intubation via direct laryngoscopy, the anesthetist must be
aware of the potential for rupturing telangiectases, which
may produce a large volume of blood loss. The bleeding can
quickly obscure and obliterate the anesthetist's view of the
airway anatomy. For this reason, direct laryngoscopy must be
relatively gentle but at the same time accomplished quickly to
avoid aspiration of blood if a telangiectatic lesion does rupture. Placement of a laryngeal mask airway should be avoided
because of the potential for rupture and hemorrhage from
telangiectatic lesions.

Because of the fragility of AVMs, the anesthetist must
strive to avoid extreme swings in this patient's blood pressure
throughout the duration of the anesthetic. The anesthetist
should also strive to reduce the inspiratory pressure during
mechanical ventilation. This may be achieved by using the
pressure-controlled ventilation and setting a relatively low
peak inspiratory pressure. In addition, the expiratory phase
should be prolonged, on the order of 1:2.5 or 1:3, to prevent
air trapping that may contribute to rupture of pulmonary
AVMs. The tidal volumes of positive pressure ventilations
should be reduced when the number of breaths per minute
increases to achieve the "calculated" minute ventilation the
patient needs. These interventions will reduce the possible
trauma to any pulmonary AVM that may be present. Appearance of blood in the endotracheal tube may indicate rupture
of a pulmonary AVM.

The anesthetist must also be alert for signs and symptoms
of a subarachnoid hemorrhage (particularly during non-neuro-
vascular surgery), which closely follow signs and symptoms of
increased intracranial pressure, such as widening pulse pressure,
bradycardia, and dilated pupils. Epidural hematoma formation
is also a significant risk during surgery. The anesthetist should
watch closely for the development of an epidural hematoma in
patients with newly demonstrated lower extremity weakness or
paralysis.

Cirrhosis in the patient with OWRS is indicative of liver
function impairment. Diminution of liver function may alter
the metabolism of several anesthesia-related drugs, such as
sodium thiopental, midazolam, opiate analgesics, and muscle

relaxants. In such events, doses of individual medications that depend heavily on the liver for metabolism/biotransformation may need to be reduced. Severe instances of arteriovenous shunting within the liver may result in the high-output form of liver failure.

Osteogenesis Imperfecta

Definition

Osteogenesis imperfecta (OI), one of the most common skeletal dysplasias, is inherited via autosomal dominant mutation(s). It is produced by defective biosynthesis of type I collagen, which results in brittle, osteoporotic bones that are easily fractured. Osteogenesis imperfecta is also known as Lobstein disease, brittle-bone disease, blue sclera disease, and fragile bone disease.

Incidence

Osteogenesis imperfecta is estimated to occur in 1:20,000 to 1:30,000 births.

Etiology

Type I collagen occurs naturally as a triple helix whose constituents are two copies of the α_1-chain and one copy of the α_2-chain. The pro–α_1-chain is encoded by the COL1A gene located on chromosome 17, whereas the pro–α_2-chain is encoded by the COL2A gene on chromosome 2. Quantitative defects of type I collagen are the result of mutations on the COL1A gene. Qualitative defects of type I collagen result from mutations of either the COL1A or COL2B gene, producing a mixture of both normal and abnormal collagen chains. The disease does not exhibit any predilection for a particular race, ethnic group, or gender.

Signs and Symptoms

- Barrel chest
- Blue sclera
- Constipation
- Defective dentition
- Fractures
- Growth retardation
- Hearing loss
- Joint laxity
- Kyphosis
- Limb deformities
- Macrocephaly
- Scoliosis
- Sweating
- Triangular face
- Wormian bones

Osteogenesis Imperfecta. A, Severe deformity of both femurs. **B,** Same individual after multiple osteotomies with telescoping medullary rod fixation. *(From Crenshaw AH, editor:* Campbell's Operative Orthopedics, *ed. 8, vol 3, St Louis, 1992, Mosby.)*

Medical Management

In the past, the primary interventions for OI consisted of deformity correction by surgical intervention, physiotherapy, orthotic support(s), and mobility-assistance devices, such as wheelchairs. As the molecular nature of this disease has become better understood, pharmacotherapy is being increasingly employed to augment bone mass and strength. Surgical intervention is kept in reserve for functional improvement.

Synthetic pyrophosphate analogues—such as bisphosphonates (particularly pamidronate)—inhibit osteoclast-mediated bone resorption. Because osteoblastic new bone formation is unopposed, cortical thickness increases, yielding stronger bone tissue. Intravenous administration of pamidronate is effective in infants, and its administration may ameliorate the natural course of the disease. In particular, pamidronate decreases the rate of fractures, increases bone mineral density, decreases bone pain, and contributes to increased height. Growth hormone may be given to act on the growth plate and stimulate osteoblast function. The patient with a quantitative collagen defect may derive somewhat greater benefit from growth hormone administration; however, the role of growth hormone has yet to be clearly delineated.

Teriparatide is a recombinant-DNA–derived form of human parathyroid hormone that has potential application in the management of OI, but that potential application has not been defined. In addition, the risk of osteosarcoma induction has thus far prevented FDA approval of administering teriparatide to children and adolescents.

Orthotics continue to occupy a limited role in the treatment of OI—as a means of stabilizing lax joints and halting progression of deformities and fractures. Walking aids, specialized wheelchairs, and home adaptation devices help the patient maintain and improve mobility. Lower limb contractures, especially when the Achilles' tendon is involved, may require soft tissue surgical correction. Painful and recurrent bone deformities are ideally treated using intramedullary stabilization devices, such as Sheffield rods, Bailey-Dubow rods, Rush pins, or Kirschner wires. Intermedullary stabilization is superior to fixation using plates/screws or solid nails because of the high risk of new fractures above or below the device and poor fixation.

Spinal deformities such as scoliosis and/or kyphosis are not amenable to application of braces for OI patients. The patient's rib cage is too fragile to withstand the requisite pressure of the "counter traction" produced by the brace. In addition, the pressure from the brace could exacerbate any chest deformity(-ies) that may be present. Surgical correction is undertaken when there is acceptably "solid" bone and more than 45 degrees of curvature in mild forms of OI or if there is 30 to 35 degrees of curvature in severe manifestations of OI.

Complications

- Adverse effects from bisphosphonate administration (acute febrile reaction, mild hypocalcemia, leukopenia, transient increased bone pain)
- Basilar invagination
- Complications of rod placement (breakage, rotational deformities, rod migration)
- Congenital heart disease
- Contractures
- Cor pulmonale
- Fractures (above or below fixation site)
- Hydrocephalus
- Hyperthermia
- Platelet dysfunction
- Respiratory depression due to brainstem compression

Anesthesia Implications

Bleeding time and coagulation parameters should be determined preoperatively. The patient with OI is prone to platelet dysfunction, and thus more susceptible to increased blood loss. It may be necessary to transfuse platelets perioperatively to lessen the degree of operative bleeding.

The patient with OI may have a relatively large head and tongue, making airway management difficult. The anesthetist must exercise great care to guard against mandibular and/or facial fractures. Neck extension during mask ventilation and direct laryngoscopy must be minimized to reduce the potential for trauma or fractures and all the concomitant untoward sequelae of cervical trauma.

This disease is characterized by "soft" or brittle bone; therefore, the patient with OI is highly prone to fractures, especially if not treated with bisphosphonates. The anesthetist should be extremely careful when using tourniquets for intravenous access, because the pressure may be sufficient to produce a fracture. In a similar fashion, the patient's arm (humerus) should be adequately padded before application of the blood pressure cuff. The anesthetist must also take great care to ensure that bony prominences and pressure points are well padded, because of the propensity for fractures resulting from seemingly very minor trauma in a patient with OI. Transfers to and from the operating room bed and stretcher must be accomplished with equal gentleness to minimize the potential for fractures.

The patient with OI should be examined visually to assess the degree of scoliosis and/or kyphosis present. Pulmonary function testing should be obtained for a patient with significant scoliosis or kyphosis to determine the degree of pulmonary encroachment the associated anomalies may have produced.

As an associated anomaly, the patient with OI is prone to hyperthermia, and so is more susceptible to a hyperthermic episode during anesthesia. Both hyperthermia without muscle rigidity and malignant hyperthermia (MH) have been documented intraoperatively in patients with OI. Therefore, the anesthetist is cautioned to treat the patient with OI in a fashion similar to that of a patient with a documented family history of MH. Known MH triggers, such as succinylcholine or halothane, should be avoided. In preparation, the anesthetist should have MH treatment medications readily available and be prepared to mechanically cool the patient before induction of general anesthesia.

Despite the above cautionary measures, no particular anesthetic technique is endorsed or recommended more than another. Regional anesthesia is acceptable; however, the nature of this disorder may make needle placement relatively complicated. Bone puncture with a spinal or epidural needle during the insertion process may result in vertebral fractures in the perioperative period as well as the pain and potential untoward sequelae attendant to vertebral fractures. In addition, interosseous injection of local anesthetic is a possibility—one that is difficult to recognize and may contribute to local anesthetic toxicity. Total intravenous anesthesia (TIVA) is an excellent choice for the conduction of anesthesia for the patient who requires general anesthesia. The choice of the medications will depend somewhat on the overall condition of the patient combined with the nature of the proposed surgical intervention.

Finally, the anesthetist must be particularly cautious when a patient with OI must be placed in any but the supine position. The patient with OI is particularly susceptible to retinal artery occlusion, and this becomes a crucial consideration when placing the patient in the prone position. In this case, hypotension, whether deliberate or incidental, should be avoided. Perioperative hypotension in the patient with OI may result in or contribute to perioperative vision loss (POVL). The anesthetist must be particularly careful to avoid external pressure on the eye globe throughout the course of the anesthesia.

Osteomalacia

Definition

Osteomalacia is a bone disease producing increasingly soft, brittle, flexible, and deformed bones because of a loss or short- age of calcium salts, or inadequate or delayed mineralization of osteoid in mature and spongy bone. Osteomalacia is often referred to as the adult form of rickets.

Incidence

The incidence of osteomalacia is reported to be less than 0.1% in developed countries. In areas with high vegetarian popula- tions, it has been reported to be as high as 15%.

Etiology

Osteomalacia is produced by a metabolic disorder for which the underlying disease needs to be diagnosed.

Causes of Rickets/Osteomalacia

- Acidosis
- Chronic renal failure
- Defective matrix synthesis
- Gastrointestinal tract inadequacy
- Generalized renal tube disorders
- Miscellaneous
- Phosphate depletion
- Primary mineralization disorders
- States of rapid bone formation with or without defect in bone resorption
- Vitamin D deficiency
- Vitamin D metabolism disorders

Signs and Symptoms

- Bowed limbs
- Craniotabes (abnormal softness of skull bone, particularly along the lambdoidal sutures)
- Genu valgum
- Joint laxity
- Mild to more pronounced scoliosis
- Muscle weakness
- Pectus carinatum
- Poor dentition
- Rachitic rosary
- Triradiate pelvis configura- tion (the pelvis radiates in three directions)

Medical Management

Vitamin D supplementation is particularly important for infants exclusively breastfed by mothers who are also deficient in vitamin D. The infant's supplementation should be at the rate of 400 International Units (IU) per day after the child has reached 2 months of age. Adults should receive vitamin D supplements daily and are strongly encouraged to increase (within reason) exposure to direct sunlight to aid the natural, *in vivo*, conversion process.

Complications

- Fractures
- Kyphosis
- Muscle cramps
- Paresthesias
- Pseudofracture
- Renal dysfunction
- Scoliosis
- Tetany

Anesthesia Implications

The anesthetist should pay particular attention to the degree of dysfunction of the patient's kidneys. Renal dysfunction may be a significant contributing factor in the development of osteomalacia. In addition, abnormal liver function may be a major contributing factor as well. Complete metabolic profiles should be obtained preoperatively and closely reviewed for indications of either kidney or liver dysfunction. Where possible, electrolyte imbalances should be corrected preoperatively.

The patient with osteomalacia is prone to develop scoliosis and/or kyphosis. A patient with either of these maladies should undergo complete pulmonary function testing preoperatively to indicate the degree of pulmonary dysfunction that may have been produced. Frequently pulmonary dysfunction develops in a restrictive form. During general anesthesia, the anesthetist should strive to reduce the peak inspiratory pressure, either by selecting lower peak pressure in the pressure-controlled volume/ventilation setting on the anesthesia ventilator or by manually ventilating the patient using the reservoir bag. The expiratory phase should also be prolonged in the patient with any restrictive lung disease to reduce the possible degree of air trapping and barotrauma. The prolonged inspiratory:expiratory (I:E) phase should be 1:2.5, 1:3—or possibly 1:3.5—depending on the severity of the restrictive pulmonary disease.

The anesthetist must be particularly attentive to the patient's positioning during surgery. Padding is extremely important for the patient with osteomalacia. Gel pads are greatly preferred to simple foam padding to prevent injury. The anesthetist must remember that the patient who is untreated or undertreated is much more susceptible to bone injury (see also Osteogenesis Imperfecta, p. 251).

Paget's Disease of the Bone

Definition

Paget's disease of the bone is a relatively common disease of middle-aged and elderly people in which there is excessive and abnormal bone remodeling. The condition results in extensively vascularized, weak, enlarged, deformed bones that are increasingly prone to subsequent complications.

Incidence

Determining the frequency of occurrence of Paget's disease is inherently imprecise because many affected people are asymptomatic. The disease is estimated to affect approximately 3% of the population 40 years of age or older. Males are more commonly affected at a ratio of 1.8:1.

Etiology

The exact etiology of Paget's disease remains unknown. Genetic and nongenetic contributions have been implicated, including factors related to viral infection, elevated parathyroid hormones, autoimmune deficiencies, connective tissue, and vascular disorders.

Signs and Symptoms

- Acetabulum protrusion
- Ataxia
- Back and neck pain
- Bone angulation and/or deformity
- Bone pain
- Bowel and bladder incontinence
- Cranial nerve palsies
- Dementia
- Dizziness
- Enlargement of skull and lower limbs
- Facial disfigurement
- Femur and long bone bowing
- Gait difficulties
- Hearing loss
- Limb paresis
- Malocclusion
- Muscle weakness
- Nausea
- Nonspecific headache
- Paresthesias
- Pathologic fractures

Paget's Disease of the Bone. Diagrammatic representation of Paget's disease of bone, demonstrating the three phases in the evolution of the disease. *(From Kumar V, Abbas AK, Fausto N: Robbins and Cotran's Pathologic Basis of Disease, ed. 7, Philadelphia, 2005, Saunders.)*

- Platybasia (also known as basilar impression: a developmental deformity of the occipital bone and upper end of the cervical spine in which the cervical spine appears to have pushed the floor of the occipital bone upward)
- Syncope
- Tibial or skull bruits
- Tinnitus
- Tooth loss
- Vertigo

Medical Management

Maintenance or improvement of muscle strength, maintaining joint range of motion and flexibility, increased endurance, and deconditioning avoidance are goals for initiation of physical therapy in the treatment of Paget's disease. Superficial heat application, transcutaneous electrical nerve stimulation, and massage are important physical therapy interventions that help reduce pain, tenderness, and tightness. Functional range-of-motion exercises are an integral incorporation to help maintain the function of major joints.

Occupational therapy is incorporated for the patient in need of training to "relearn" the performance of basic activities of daily life. Involving two occupational therapists in conjunction with physical therapy may strengthen the patient's independence, safety, and mobility and can result in better maintenance or improvement of muscle strength.

Indications for Pharmacotherapy in the Patient with Paget's Disease of the Bone

- Anticipated joint arthroplasty
- Bone pain
- Bony deformities
- Cardiac complications
- Hypercalcemia or hypercalciuria
- Neurologic complications
- Osteolytic lesions
- Prevention of future complications
- Serum alkaline or urine hydroxyproline more than twice the upper reference range
- Skull or spine disease
- Weight-bearing bone involvement

P

Complications

- Angioid streaks of the retina
- Autonomic hyperreflexia
- Calcific aortic stenosis
- Cranial nerve palsies
- Degenerative joint disease
- High-output cardiac failure
- Hydrocephalus
- Left ventricular hypertrophy
- Pagetic sarcoma
- Pathologic fractures
- Platybasia
- Spastic quadriplegia
- Spinal cord compression
- Stress fractures

Anesthesia Implications

Securing the airway is always a concern for the anesthetist. That concern is increased for a patient with Paget's disease of the bone. The characteristic bony fragility may be displayed in the patient's facial bones, particularly the maxillae or mandible. Application of excess force during mask ventilation may produce significant injury. The patient with Paget's disease is also prone to cervical instability and may become paraplegic with manipulation or head positioning for mask ventilation and/or intubation. The anesthetist must strive to maintain head neutrality throughout the process of direct laryngoscopy.

Positioning the patient requires more patience and indulgence than usual. Whenever feasible, the patient should be allowed or encouraged to position himself or herself to afford as much comfort as possible. Bony prominences and pressure points should be amply padded. Gel pads are preferable to foam padding because they disperse pressure more effectively while providing some measure of support.

Regional anesthesia may be appropriate, especially for total joint arthroplasty procedures. However, the spine should be examined radiographically to help the anesthetist avoid placing the needle into or through pathologic bone or injecting the local anesthetic into the same pathologic bone, which can result in a greater degree of toxic reaction.

The patient with Paget's disease is frequently treated with nonsteroidal anti-inflammatory drugs (NSAIDs). The patient should be instructed to terminate the use of these drugs 10 days before elective surgery, but the anesthetist should evaluate the patient's bleeding times and platelet function capabilities immediately preoperatively. The anesthetist should also be prepared for blood loss volumes in excess of the "usual and customary" for a given surgical procedure, particularly when the procedure involves the patient's bones. In addition, the anesthetist should anticipate longer surgical/operative times when procedures involving instrumentation must be performed on sclerotic bone, which may also exacerbate the amount of blood loss the patient will incur. Massive blood transfusions should be anticipated and prepared for when the lower extremities are the surgical site.

The patient with kyphosis should have his or her pulmonary function evaluated before the day of surgery. The anesthetist and the patient should discuss the potential need for post-operative ventilatory support, particularly for a patient with significantly decreased pulmonary reserves and/or an airway that is difficult to secure.

If the patient has a spinal cord lesion, the anesthetist should be prepared to treat the sequelae associated with autonomic hyperreflexia (see p. 36). The anesthetist must be prepared to treat either hypotension or hypertension at a moment's notice.

P

Pemphigoid/Pemphigus

Definition

Pemphoigoid and pemphigus are a group of chronic, autoimmune blistering diseases that are classified depending on the tissue predominately involved. Cicatricial pemphigoid (CP) predominately affects the mucous membranes, such as the conjunctiva, buccal membrates, and oropharynx, whereas bullous pemphigoid (BP) predominately affects the skin.

Pemphigoid/Pemphigus Variants	
Pemphigoid	**Pemphigus**
• Bullous pemphigoid	• Erythematous pemphigus
• Cicatricial pemphigoid	• Pemphigus foliaceous
	• Pemphigus vegetans
	• Pemphigus vulgaris

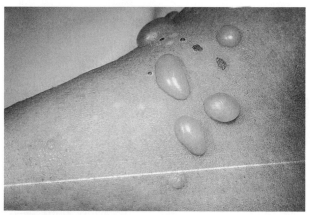

Pemphigoid/Pemphigus. Bullous pemphigoid; close-up of tense bullae. *(From Swartz MH:* Textbook of Physical Diagnosis: History and Examination, *ed. 5, Philadelphia, 2006, Saunders.)*

P

Incidence

The exact incidence of pemphigoid/pemphigus is not known.

Etiology

In CP, basement membrane zone target antigens, bullous pemphigoid antigen Z (BPAGZ), and epiligrin are attacked by autoantibodies.

In BP, the true cause is unknown; however, several possible contributing factors have been proposed, including immunogenetics, age, epitope spreading, complement activation, and chemokines.

Signs and Symptoms

Cicatricial Pemphigoid

- Alopecia from scalp erosions
- Ankyloblepharon
- Conjunctivitis
- Corneal epithelium keratinization
- Corneal sulcus shortening
- Dysphagia
- Epistaxis
- Erosions of the genitelia (clitoris, labia, glans, penile shaft)
- Hoarseness
- Nasal crusting
- Ocular dryness
- Pruritus
- Recurrent, painful erosions of the mouth, particularly the gingivae, palate, and buccal mucosa
- Severe ocular inflammation (unilateral or bilateral) after eye surgery
- Symblepharon
- Synechiae

Bullous Pemphigoid

- Dysphagia
- Exfoliative erythroderma
- Generalized atopic dermatitis
- Generalized bullous formation on palms and/or soles
- Psoriasis-like skin appearance
- Tense bullae (particularly on flexible skin surfaces)
- Urticarial or erythematous-based small, tense blisters (vesicular form)
- Vegetating plaques in intertriginous skin areas (vegetative form)

P

Medical Management

Therapeutic measures for either CP or BP are directed toward decreasing formation of blisters, promoting healing of blisters and/or erosions, and determining the minimal effective dose to control the disease processes. Therapeutic measures must be individualized and take into account any preexisting condition(s) the patient may have.

Bullae and/or erosions should be gently cleaned on a daily basis. Compresses, topical agents that promote wound healing, and/or biologic dressings may be applied to minimize trauma, hasten healing, and reduce scarring.

The patient with CP may need ongoing ophthalmic evaluation because of the high degree of involvement of the eyes. Ablation of ingrown eyelashes may be necessary to prevent further damage to the eyes. The mucosal membranes of the pharynx and/or trachea may produce significant respiratory compromise and require tracheostomy. Scarring of the esophagus may necessitate repeated dilation procedures.

Complications

- Adrenal suppression
- Ankyloblepharon
- Blindness
- Bone marrow suppression
- Corneal keratinization
- Esophageal strictures/ stenosis
- Fornices foreshortening
- Fractures
- Growth retardation
- Infection (localized or systemic)
- Malignancy
- Osteoporosis
- Symblepharon
- Synechiae
- Tracheal stenosis
- Trichiasis
- Visual acuity loss

Anesthesia Implications

Airway management is always a strong concern for the anesthetist and is magnified for patients with CP. Blister formation occurs easily in the patient with CP, even with relatively insignificant trauma, such as while eating food that is hard (e.g., chips, raw vegetables). As a result, airway compromise may be present when the patient presents to the operating room. Direct laryngoscopy and other instrumentation should be avoided if possible, but when unavoidable, should be undertaken with great caution. The anesthetist should expect to produce blisters during direct laryngoscopy. In addition, the airway should be secured with a smaller than usual endotracheal tube to reduce the degree of trauma to the vocal cords and trachea. Because of the friction involved in the placement procedure, the laryngeal mask airway should be avoided in the patient with pemphigoid/pemphigus.

As an autoimmune disease, treatment may consist of immunsuppression agents. Bone marrow toxicity and extensive hepatic effects may be present in the patient with pemphigoid. Bone marrow toxicity may significantly alter the patient's hematopoiesis perioperatively. Liver function and complete blood count levels should be evaluated preoperatively. The anesthetist should be aware that the patient with pemphigoid may be chronically dehydrated due to lack of oral intake as the result of pain from oral or oropharyngeal blisters and/or erosions. Therefore hemoglobin and hematocrit values may be artificially "normal" or even appear to be elevated. In addition, the self-restriction of nutrition and fluids as the result of the pain may also result in significant alterations in the electrolyte concentrations. Significant electrolyte losses may result from rupture and drainage of the numerous blisters the patient may have.

A patient with either form of pemphigoid is likely to be receiving corticosteroid medications as a part of the immunosuppression therapy. The patient should receive a perioperative dose of corticosteroid; an exacerbation of the disease is possible should the corticosteroid coverage be omitted.

▶ Polyarteritis Nodosa

Definition

Polyarteritis nodosa (PAN) is a rare form of systemic necrotizing vasculitis that primarily affects small and medium-sized arteries without glomerulonephritis or vasculitis in the arterioles, capillaries, or venules.

Incidence

In the United States the incidence of PAN is 3:100,000 to 4.5:100,000 per year. Internationally the incidence is 1.8:100,000 to 6.3:100,000 per year, except in populations with endemic hepatitis B, where the incidence of PAN can reach 7.7:100,000. There is no observed racial predilection, and males are more frequently affected by a ratio of 1.6:1. The onset usually occurs between 40 and 60 years of age.

Etiology

An immune response is the suspected cause of PAN. About 30% of patients with PAN test positive for the hepatitis B surface antigen. The hepatitis B antigen aggregates with circulating hepatitis B antibodies in the serum and produces vascular lesions.

Signs and Symptoms

- Abdominal pain
- Arthralgia
- Arthritis
- Bleeding
- Bowel infarction
- Bowel perforation
- Cholecystitis
- Congestive heart failure
- Cutaneous infarcts
- Cutaneous neuropathy
- Distal polyneuropathy
- Encephalopathy
- Fever
- Headache
- Hepatic infarction
- Hypertension
- Livedo reticularis (a vascular response to various disorders caused by dilation of the subpapillary venous plexus as a result of increased blood viscosity

P

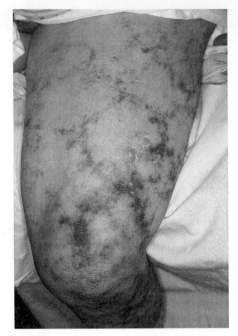

Polyarteritis Nodosa. Cutaneous polyarteritis nodosa as manifested by a livedo pattern with purpuric and necrotic lesions. *(From Callen JP, et al: Dermatological Signs of Internal Disease, ed 3, Philadelphia, 2003, Saunders.)*

which changes the blood vessels delaying blood flow away from the skin)
- Malaise
- Mononeuritis multiplex
- Myalgia
- Myelopathy
- Myocardial infarction
- Nausea
- Nodules
- Pancreatic infarction
- Pericarditis
- Purpura
- Rash
- Raynaud's phenomenon
- Renal failure
- Seizures, cerebral ischemia
- Testicular or ovarian pain
- Vomiting
- Weakness
- Weight loss

Medical Management

The standard treatment for the patient with idiopathic PAN, as well as those with more severe manifestations of the disease, is administration of corticosteroids combined with cyclophosphamide. The patient whose PAN is identified with hepatitis B may be treated with a regimen that includes plasmapheresis and/or antiviral medications. Immunomodulation therapy seems to work well, but the therapeutic response is optimized when a corticosteroid, such as prednisone, is combined with cyclophosphamide rather than administered alone. Surgical intervention may be limited to microembolization of a cerebral aneurysm when this is determined to be appropriate.

Complications

- Bowel infarction
- Encephalopathy
- Gastrointestinal bleeding
- Heart failure
- Myelopathy
- Myocardial infarction
- Pericarditis
- Peripheral neuropathy
- Renal failure
- Stroke

Anesthesia Implications

Lesions of PAN frequently occur in the kidneys, lungs, heart, brain, gastrointestinal tract, liver, adrenal glands, testes, ovaries, and peripheral nerves. The vessels of these organs, in particular, are vulnerable to weakening and dilation. Rupture of lesions of these organs can result in significant blood loss.

On presentation to the operating room, the patient with PAN is generally in serious condition. Bowel perforation may be the precipitating event, requiring surgical intervention. Rapid sequence induction of anesthesia is preferred because of the higher potential for aspiration secondary to gastrointestinal manifestations of the disease process. The patient's blood pressure should be closely monitored and any hypertensive episode treated without delay because of the potential for untoward cerebral sequelae, such as subdural bleeding or aneurysm rupture.

The airway of the patient with PAN may be unexpectedly difficult to secure. Patients with PAN have been documented to have episodes of acute pharyngeal edema encompassing the uvula and other peripharyngeal structures. Instrumentation for intubation should be undertaken with great caution and care, and may be best attempted by a senior or veteran anesthetist. The anesthetist may have only a single opportunity to secure this patient's airway. The difficult airway cart should be immediately at hand, including the fiberoptic bronchoscope.

It may be necessary to enlist a surgeon to surgically secure the patient's airway.

The anesthetist should strive to maintain normothermia for this patient. The patient with PAN is prone to Raynaud's phenomenon. The anesthetist should be sure to warm intravenous fluids as well as provide external warming using a forced-air system.

P

Portal Hypertension

Definition

Portal hypertension is the presence within the portal circulation of a pressure gradient of 12 mm Hg or higher. This malady is associated with numerous conditions as listed in the box below.

Conditions Associated with Portal Hypertension

- Family history of hemochromatosis or Wilson's disease (see p. 355)
- History of alcohol abuse
- History of blood transfusions and/or intravenous drug use (hepatitis B and/or C)
- History of jaundice
- Pruritus

Incidence

The frequency of occurrence of portal hypertension is not known.

Etiology

Development of portal hypertension can result from many causes, generally classified as prehepatic, intrahepatic (presinusoidal), intrahepatic (sinusoidal and/or postsinusoidal), and posthepatic.

Signs and Symptoms

- Altered sleep patterns
- Ascites
- Asterixis
- Clubbing of digits
- Distended abdominal wall veins (caput medusae)
- Dupuytren's contracture
- Esophageal varices
- Gynecomastia
- Hematochezia
- Hepatic encephalopathy
- Hepatorenal syndrome
- Increased irritability
- Increasing abdominal girth

P

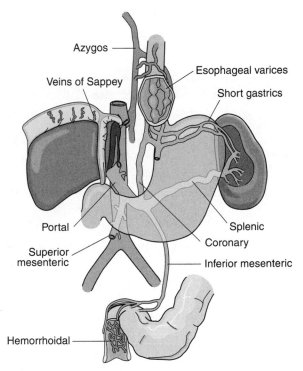

Portal Hypertension. Varices related to portal hypertension. Portal vein, its major tributaries, and the most important shunts (collateral veins) between the portal and caval systems. *(From Monahan FD, et al:* Phipps' Medical-Surgical Nursing: Health and Illness Persepectives, *ed. 8, St Louis, 2007, Mosby.)*

Causes of Portal Hypertension

Intrahepatic (Presinusoidal)
- Early schistosomiasis
- Hepatic metastasis
- Idiopathic portal hypertension
- Myeloproliferative disease
- Nodular regenerative hyperplasia
- Polycystic disease
- Primary biliary cirrhosis

Intrahepatic (Sinusoidal and/ or Postsinusoidal)
- Acute alcoholic hepatitis
- Acute and fulminant hepatitis
- Advanced idiopathic portal hypertension
- Advanced primary biliary cirrhosis
- Advanced schistosomiasis
- Budd-Chiari syndrome (see p. 59)
- Congenital hepatic fibrosis
- Hepatic cirrhosis

- Peliosis hepatis
- Veno-occlusive disease
- Vitamin A toxicity

Posthepatic
- Arterial-portal venous fistula
- Budd-Chiari syndrome (see p. 59)
- Constrictive pericarditis
- Increased portal blood flow
- Increased splenic blood flow
- Inferior vena cava obstruction
- Right-sided heart failure
- Tricuspid regurgitation

Prehepatic
- Congenital atresia
- Portal vein stenosis
- Portal vein thrombosis
- Splanchnic arteriovenous fistula
- Splenic vein thrombosis

- Jaundice
- Lethargy
- Muscle wasting
- Palmar erythema
- Rectal varices

- Spider angiomas
- Splenomegaly
- Spontaneous bacterial peritonitis (SBP)
- Testicular atrophy

Medical Management

Medical care for the patient with portal hypertension is aimed at correcting the underlying cause/disease. Treatment regimens may be categorized as emergent, primary prophylactic, and elective.

Emergent treatment is initiated for the patient presenting with bleeding esophageal varices. Replacement of lost blood volume is the initial treatment measure, with the goal to return the patient's hematocrit to about a 25% to 30% concentration. Replacement measures must avoid overexpanding the intravascular volume, especially the volume of the varices, to reduce the potential for continued and/or recurrent bleeding.

P

The source of the bleeding should be determined as quickly as possible.

Pharmacologic treatment may include various compounds, such as vasopressin or octreotide, which act to reduce portal blood flow and/or pressure. Intravenous nitrates are frequently administered in conjunction with vasopressin to significantly improve the latter's efficacy. Emergent treatment may also include endoscopic sclerotherapy injection, endoscopic variceal ligation, or balloon-tube tamponade (in the event of massive hemorrhage).

Primary prophylaxis is typically employed in a patient considered at high risk for bleeding whether because of severe liver failure, the presence of large varices, or red wale markings on the varices. Prophylactic treatment regimens may entail the administration of β-blocking medications to reduce portal and collateral blood flow. Vasodilators, such as isosorbide mononitrate, may be administered to reduce the high venous pressure gradient and they may reduce esophageal variceal pressure as well.

Sclerotherapy or variceal ligation may be undertaken to prevent hemorrhage. Randomized, controlled clinical trials of sclerotherapy as a primary prophylactic measure have yielded divergent results. As a result, prophylactic sclerotherapy is considered to have no role as a primary prophylactic intervention. Endoscopic ligation has demonstrated greater effectiveness in prevention of initial variceal bleeding. The efficacy demonstrated is similar to results achieved by administration of β-blocking medications.

Surgical interventions are categorized as decompression shunts, devascularization procedures, or liver transplantation. Decompressive shunting is achieved with total portal systemic shunting, partial portal systemic shunting, or other selective shunting, such as the distal splenorenal shunt. Devascularization procedures include splenectomy, gastroesophageal devascularization, or esophageal transection. Liver transplantation is the ultimate procedure to alleviate portal hypertension, recurrent variceal hemorrhage, ascites, and encephalopathy because it fully restores liver function.

Complications

- Ascites
- Bronchial aspiration
- Gastrointestinal varices
- Hepatic encephalopathy
- Hepatorenal syndrome
- Renal failure
- Subacute bacterial peritonitis
- Systemic infection
- Variceal hemorrhage

Anesthesia Implications

Portal hypertension is most commonly a result of significant liver dysfunction, such as cirrhosis or failure. This patient's clotting ability is questionable at best and should be assessed immediately preoperatively if at all possible. Protein synthesis, specifically production of clotting factors, may be significantly altered by liver dysfunction. Before invasive procedures on the patient with portal hypertension, administration of vitamin K and/or transfusion with fresh frozen plasma may be necessary. If laboratory data indicate the need for these therapeutic measures, they should be administered preoperatively.

Chronic liver failure often incurs chronic steroid administration. The steroid administration should be maintained on the regular schedule during the perioperative period; the dosage may need to be increased. Administration of histamine (H_2)-antagonists may help reduce the potential for gastrointestinal bleeding.

Because of the high association of portal hypertension with significant liver dysfunction or failure, drug metabolism will likely be prolonged. Most anesthesia-related drugs, from muscle relaxants to opioids to benzodiazepines to hypnotics, depend on hepatic metabolism for elimination. These medications' dosages will need to be reduced to lessen the metabolic load on the already dysfunctional liver. Where muscle relaxation is necessary, the more appropriate choice would be atracurium or *cis*-atracurium. Mivacurium may not be appropriate because of the potentially low pseudocholinesterase concentrations the patient with portal hypertension may have. Due to this same cause, succinylcholine should be avoided as well.

P

Pulmonary Alveolar Proteinosis

Definition

Pulmonary alveolar proteinosis (PAP) is a rare lung disease characterized by filling of the distal alveoli with endogenous proteinaceous or floccular material derived from surfactant phospholipids and protein components. This disease presents in two forms: primary (idiopathic) or secondary (resulting from infection, hematologic malignancy(ies) or inhalation of a foreign substance).

Incidence

The incidence of PAP is estimated to be 1:100,000. Males are affected more often by a ratio of 4:1.

Etiology

The etiology of primary PAP is still not known. Secondary PAP is associated with several processes, which lends credence to a causal relationship. The associated processes include inhalation of inorganic/mineral dusts (e.g., silica, titanium oxide, aluminum) or organic materials (e.g., insecticides); hematologic malignancy(ies); myeloid, lysinuric protein intolerance, or HIV infection.

Signs and Symptoms

- Clubbing of digits
- Cor pulmonale (rare)
- Cyanosis (rare)
- Fatigue
- Fine end-inspiratory crackles
- Hemoptysis (rare)
- Intermittent low-grade fever
- Intermittent night sweats
- Malaise
- Persistent dry cough
- Pleuritic chest pain
- Progressive dyspnea
- Pulmonary hypertension
- Weight loss

Medical Management

Medical care of the patient with primary PAP is predicated on the presence or absence of a coexisting infection, the extensiveness of progression of the disease, as well as the degree of physiologic impairment. In the past, treatment consisted of administration of corticosteroids, aerosolized mucolytics, and aerosolized proteinases, but success in this treatment regimen was limited.

The current standard of care for treating the patient with PAP is whole-lung lavage to mechanically remove the accumulated lipoproteinaceous materials. Whole-lung lavage requires general anesthesia via a double-lumen endobronchial tube. Placement of the tube makes it possible to lavage one lung while ventilating the other. Both lungs are first ventilated for several minutes with 100% oxygen. One lung is then isolated and lavaged with 0.9% isotonic saline solution. The saline remains in the lung for a few minutes and is suctioned out as completely as possible. The treated lung is allowed to recover, usually for a period of several days, after which general anesthesia is employed and the process repeated for the other lung.

Complications

- Cor pulmonale
- Lung infections
- Pulmonary fibrosis

Anesthesia Implications

The patient should have pulmonary function testing (PFT) done before the administration of any proposed anesthetic, whether for whole-lung lavage or any other surgical intervention. The results of the PFTs can identify a restrictive lung disease with reduced lung volumes, altered lung compliance, and/or decreased diffusing capacity. The anesthetist should strive to keep peak inspiratory pressures as low as possible, which can be aided by selection of the pressure-controlled ventilation mode on many newer anesthesia machines. In addition, the patient should be placed on a prolonged expiratory phase during ventilation, on the order of 1:2.5 or 1:3. Both measures are aimed at maximizing the patient's gas exchange while limiting or preventing air trapping and potential lung injury.

The patient scheduled for whole-lung lavage requires a double-lumen endobronchial tube. Preoxygenation should be longer than usual because of the restrictive nature of PAP as well as the longer time needed, generally, for placement and confirmation of tube placement, along with the increased pulmonary shunting typically found in PAP patients.

The patient with PAP should have an arterial pressure line inserted before the proposed procedure. Serial blood gas analysis samples should obtained, beginning preoperatively, to establish the patient's baseline, and thereafter to mark the progress of the treatment and ventilatory adequacy.

The patient undergoing whole-lung lavage may benefit from the use of total intravenous anesthesia (TIVA), in part because of the reduced lung area that will be available for the provision of an inhalational agent. Whole-lung lavage may require several hours to complete. The patient should receive 100% oxygen throughout the procedure. Conventional inhalational anesthesia remains a viable and safe method for provision of anesthesia, just as would be the case for anesthesia for a patient undergoing pneumonectomy or lobectomy.

Whole-lung lavage requires that large volumes of isotonic saline solution be placed into a lung over the course of several hours. Ideally the irrigation solution used should be warmed to body temperature or slightly higher before instillation. These fluids may cool in the operating room environment to considerably lower than body temperature. Therefore the patient's body core temperature should be closely followed because of the risk of hypothermia. However, the esophageal temperature probe may give a false positive of normothermia or hypothermia because the temperature recorded may more closely reflect that of the irrigation fluid than that of the patient. As a result, the patient's temperature should also be measured at other sites, using instruments such as a nasopharyngeal or a rectal temperature probe, or taking blood temperature from the central circulation. Because of the absorbing and diffusing capabilities of the lungs, the anesthetist must be alert to the amount of irrigation solution instilled compared to the volume that is suctioned out. The large volumes of fluid used in the procedure can cause a fluid volume overload and symptoms similar to those of congestive heart failure. Even when more fluid is removed than instilled, the anesthetist must remember that this difference owes in large part to the proteinaceous material being removed and that the potential for fluid overload remains very real.

On completion of the procedure, the patient with PAP should remain intubated until lung function demonstrates adequate recovery. Adequacy of recovery may be assessed by improved lung compliance at a level near to or even greater than the preoperative baseline measurement. An acceptable level of arterial oxygen saturation via arterial blood gas analysis is also a criterion for adequate recovery. Postoperatively, possibly while awaiting the second lung lavage, the patient with PAP should be encouraged to use incentive spirometry to maintain lung compliance improvements, continue the re-expansion process, and lessen atelectasis.

Pulmonary Arteriovenous Fistula

Definition

Pulmonary arteriovenous fistula (PAVF) is an abnormal communication between the pulmonary arteries and vein. It is typically a congenital anomaly, but may also develop as the result of a number of acquired conditions/diseases. The end result of this communication is a right-to-left shunt.

Conditions Associated with Pulmonary Arteriovenous Fistula Formation
• Actinomycosis
• Fanconi syndrome (see p. 132)
• Hepatic cirrhosis
• Metastatic thyroid carcinoma
• Mitral stenosis
• Schistosomiasis
• Trauma

Incidence

The exact frequency has not been documented because PAVFs have not been carefully studied. In adults PAVF seems to occur more frequently in females than in males by almost a 2:1 ratio; among newborns, males are more frequently affected.

Etiology

The exact cause of PAVF has not been demonstrated. One theory suggests that a defect resulting in dilation of thin capillary sacs occurs in the terminal arterial loop. A different theory suggests the cause may be an incomplete resorption of the vascular septa separating the arterial and venous plexus that would usually anastomose during fetal development. Still another theory points to development of small PAVFs resulting from failure of capillary development during fetal growth.

P

Signs and Symptoms

- Anemia
- Chest pain
- Congestive heart failure
- Cough
- Cyanosis
- Diplopia
- Dizziness
- Dysarthria
- Dyspnea
- Epistaxis
- Hemoptysis
- Migraine headache
- Syncope
- Tinnitus
- Vertigo

Medical Management

Pharmacologic therapy is not a part of the standard of care for treating PAVF. However, the patient with PAVF definitely needs prophylactic antibiotic therapy before undergoing any dental or surgical procedures. Sporadic reports have advocated use of danazol, octreotide, desmopressin, or aminocaproic acid to treat epistaxis or gastrointestinal hemorrhage in patients with PAVF. The definitive treatment for PAVF is either therapeutic embolization or surgical resection.

Indications for Embolotherapy or Surgical Resection to Treat Pulmonary Arteriovenous Fistula

- Feeding vessels reach circumferences of 3 mm or larger
- Paradoxic embolization
- Progressive lesion enlargement
- Systemic hypoxemia

Complications

- Anemia
- Brain abscess
- Cerebral vascular accident
- Congestive heart failure
- Hemothorax
- Hypoxemia
- Infectious endocarditis
- Massive hemoptysis
- Migraine headache
- Orthodeoxia
- Polycythemia
- Pulmonary hypertension
- Seizure
- Transient ischemic attack

P

Complications from Therapeutic Embolization

- Air embolism
- Blood vessel rupture
- Bradydysrhythmia
- Device migration
- Pulmonary infarction
- Tachydysrhythmia
- Vascular occlusion

Anesthesia Implications

The anesthetist has two major concerns when caring for the patient with PAVF. The first involves gas exchange, and the second involves systemic emboli formation. Problems with gas exchange occur because PAVF is a right-to-left shunting of blood, which mixes the deoxygenated blood with oxygenated blood and contributes to the distribution of that mixture throughout the systemic circulation. The anesthetist's goal is to reduce the flow through the PAVF, in effect, to isolate the fistula to the extent possible. The relative isolation of the fistula can be enhanced by positioning the patient so that the PAVF is not in a dependent position, which will reduce the proportion of blood flow through the fistula, thus reducing the amount of right-to-left shunting and improving oxygenation. The anesthetist should also strive to minimize physiologic factors such as hypoxia and hypercarbia, acidosis, hypothermia, and hyperinflation of the lungs, which increase pulmonary vascular resistance and thus exacerbate the degree of right-to-left shunting via the PAVF. Positive end-expiratory pressure (PEEP) should not be used because it essentially redistributes blood flow in the lungs, thus increasing blood flow through the PAVF and exacerbating the degree of right-to-left shunting.

The anesthetist must realize that the right-to-left shunting via the PAVF bypasses the filtration process provided by the pulmonary vascular tree. As a result, any particulate or inclusion (e.g., air embolus, thrombus) may be shunted into the systemic circulation and produce potentially harmful or fatal consequences, such as a stroke or myocardial infarction. The anesthetist must be meticulous in flushing/removing air from the intravenous tubing, particularly from injection ports and stopcocks.

Resection of the PAVF can result in significant blood loss during surgery. The anesthetist should obtain the best possible intravenous access preoperatively; bilateral large-bore peripheral catheters or, preferably, central venous access plus a single large-bore peripheral intravenous line are indicated. The anesthetist must ensure the capability of rapid infusion of crystalloids, colloids, and/or blood or blood products in anticipation of intraoperative blood losses. Also, because of the potentially rapid fluid shifts involved with resection of the PAVF, the anesthetist should insert an arterial pressure catheter to closely monitor the patient's blood pressure.

Finally, the anesthetist should use a double-lumen endobronchial tube. The double-lumen tube will provide two advantages: (1) exposure of the surgical site is greatly enhanced, and (2) isolation of the operative lung protects the nonoperative lung from aspiration of blood during the surgical procedure and the reduced air exchange that results.

P

Pulmonary Hemosiderosis

Definition

Pulmonary hemosiderosis is repeated or chronic episodes of intra-alveolar bleeding resulting in iron accumulation (hemosiderin) in alveolar macrophages, culminating in pulmonary fibrosis and severe anemia. It can occur as either a primary or secondary disease process.

Incidence

The rate of occurrence of pulmonary hemosiderosis is low but the disease is well recognized. Exact figures of the incidence of pulmonary hemosiderosis have not been reported. In patients younger than 10 years of age, there is a 1:1 male to female ratio, but after 10 years of age, it increases to a 2:1 male to female ratio.

Etiology

Primary pulmonary hemosiderosis has three established variants:
1. Associated with antiglomerular basement membrane (Goodpasture syndrome, see p. 152)
2. Associated with hypersensitivity to cow's milk proteins (Heiner syndrome)
3. Idiopathic pulmonary hemosiderosis

The patient with idiopathic pulmonary hemosiderosis has a poor prognosis; the mean survival after diagnosis is generally 2.5 to 5 years. Secondary pulmonary hemosiderosis may develop as the result of a number of systemic disorders.

Causes of Secondary Hemosiderosis	
Congenital/Acquired Cardiopulmonary Anomalies • Bronchogenic cyst • Congenital arteriovenous fistula • Congenital pulmonary vein stenosis • Eisenmenger syndrome (see p. 110)	• Left ventricular failure • Mitral valve stenosis • Pulmonary arterial stenosis • Pulmonary embolism • Pulmonary sequestration • Pulmonic valve stenosis • Tetralogy of Fallot

Causes of Secondary Hemosiderosis—cont'd

Drugs
- Cocaine
- Penicillamine

Environmental Molds
- Congenital hyperammonemia
- Memroniella echinata

Immunologic Disorders
- Allergic bronchopulmonary aspergillosis
- Henoch-Schönlein purpura
- Immune complex mediated glomerulonephritis
- Periarteritis nodosa
- Pulmonary alveolar proteinosis
- Satra
- Systemic lupus erythematosus (see p. 335)
- Wegener's granulomatosis (see p. 345)

Infections
- Bacterial pneumonia
- Bronchiectasis
- Disseminated intravascular coagulation (DIC)
- Pulmonary abscess
- Sepsis

Neoplasms
- Metastatic lesions (sarcoma, Wilms' tumor, osteogenic sarcoma)
- Primary bronchial tumors (adenoma, carcinoid, sarcoma, hemangioma, angioma)

Miscellaneous Causes
- Congenital hyperammonemia
- Pulmonary alveolar proteinosis
- Pulmonary trauma
- Retained foreign body

Signs and Symptoms

- Chronic fatigue
- Chronic rhinitis
- Clubbing of digits
- Cough
- Crackles
- Cyanosis
- Diffuse pulmonary infiltrates
- Dyspnea
- Fever
- Frank respiratory failure
- Growth failure
- Hemoptysis
- Hypoxia
- Iron deficient anemia
- Pallor
- Poor weight gain
- Recurrent cough
- Recurrent otitis media
- Severe exercise limitation
- Tachypnea
- Wheezing

Medical Management

For medical management interventions associated with Goodpasture syndrome, see p. 152.

In general, pulmonary hemosiderosis is treated with oxygen supplementation and blood transfusion in cases of severe anemia and/or shock. Severe pulmonary manifestations may include excessive secretions and bronchospasm.

Intubation and mechanical ventilation may be necessary for the patient with severe pulmonary hemorrhage.

Heiner syndrome is best treated by completely eliminating cow's milk from the patient's diet, along with other dairy products.

The patient with secondary pulmonary hemosiderosis may receive the same general treatment measures described above. Additionally, the treatment regimen focuses primarily on the systemic disorder/disease from which the pulmonary hemosiderosis has emerged.

There are no specific surgical interventions indicated in the treatment of pulmonary hemosiderosis.

Complications

- Cor pulmonale
- Pulmonary fibrosis
- Pulmonary hemorrhage
- Pulmonary hypertension
- Respiratory failure

Anesthesia Implications

As the name of the disorder implies, the primary organs affected are the lungs. Serial chest x-rays may demonstrate transient perihilar and basilar infiltrates that produce a mottled appearance.

The patient should be evaluated preoperatively for iron deficiency anemia. Preoperative transfusion(s) should be based on the patient's compensatory abilities and anticipated blood loss during the perioperative period.

The pulmonary effects combined with the anemia conspire to reduce the oxygen-carrying capacity as well as gas exchange in general. Prudence dictates obtaining an arterial blood gas sample preoperatively to assess the pulmonary effects of the disease.

Because of the need to deliver good pulmonary toilet, the anesthetist should insert a larger than usual endotracheal tube.

Pulmonary fibrosis, to the degree present, produces a pattern of restrictive lung disease. Prolonging the inspiratory phase, minimizing the inspiratory pressure, and lengthening the expiratory phase will reduce the possibility of barotraumas. These parameters may be accomplished in one of two ways:

1. Possibly the simpler option would be to select pressure-controlled ventilation with a lower peak inspiratory pressure setting; this option is available on many newer models of anesthesia machines.
2. If the anesthetist does not have access to a newer model anesthesia machine, manual ventilation using the reservoir bag is an option, but because of the possibility of anesthetist fatigue, it is probably best to use this method only when the proposed procedure is estimated to require 1 hour or less.

In addition to inspiratory pressure reduction, the inspiratory:expiratory (I:E) ratio should be prolonged, possibly to 1:2.5, 1:3, or 1:3.5, to allow for completion of expiration and reduce air trapping and possible barotrauma as well. Postoperative ventilatory support should be anticipated, particularly in cases of pulmonary hemorrhage. Depending on the degree of pulmonary hemorrhage, the anesthetist may need to consider additional invasive monitoring, such as direct arterial pressure and central venous pressure, to guide fluid resuscitation and/or transfusion therapy.

Pyelonephritis

Definition

Pyelonephritis is a potentially organ-threatening, fatal inflammation of the kidney and renal pelvis secondary to a bacterial infection that begins in the interstitial tissues and rapidly extends to involve the renal tubules and glomeruli, culminating in the renal blood vessels.

Incidence

Approximately 250,000 cases of pyeolonephritis occur each year in the United States. About 192,000 of these cases require hospitalization. There have been no discernable racial or ethnic predilections, but females strongly outnumber males.

Etiology

The root cause of pyelonephritis is bacterial infection/invasion of the kidney parenchyma (see box below). Finding the cause of pyelonephritis requires determining the following: (1) which pathogens are typically cultured and their frequency; (2) whether the urinary tract infection is complicated; and (3) which pathogenic organism is involved in the complicated urinary tract infection. A complicated urinary tract infection (UTI) is defined as one occurring along with an additional factor that reduces the efficacy of antimicrobial therapy and leads to therapy failure, relapses, or persistence of infection.

Causative Organisms in Pyelonephritis

- Citrobacter species
- Coagulase-negative Staphylococci
- Enterobacter species
- Enterococci
- *Escherichia coli*
- Group B Streptococci
- Klebsiella species
- *Proteus mirabilis*
- *Pseudomonas aeruginosa*
- *Staphylococcus aureus*

P

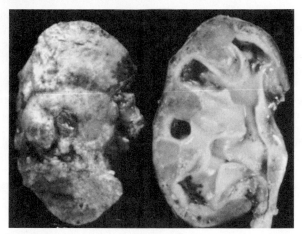

Pyelonephritis. Chronic pyelonephritis. The surface (left) is irregularly scarred. The cut section (right) reveals characteristic dilation and blunting of calyces. *(From Kumar V, Abbas AK, Fausto N: Robbins and Cotran's Pathologic Basis of Disease, ed. 7, Philadelphia, 2005, Saunders.)*

Signs and Symptoms

- Anorexia
- Chills
- Fever (sometimes)
- Malaise
- Mild-to-moderate or severe pain
- Nausea
- Rigor
- Tachycardia
- Unilateral or bilateral flank pain
- Vomiting

Medical Management

The mainstay of medical care of the patient with pyelonephritis is supportive. It consists of rest, antipyretics, analgesics (oral or parenteral), antiemetics (oral or parenteral), dysuric relief using urinary tract analgesics, and oral or parenteral fluid to maintain proper hydration. However, these palliative measures may not be sufficient. Hospitalization may become necessary to intensify treatment because of the inability to tolerate oral intake, poor treatment compliance, poor treatment follow-up, unstable vital signs, increasing severity of signs and symptoms, pregnancy, and co-morbidity problems (e.g., diabetes mellitus, an acquired immunodeficiency). Patient treatment should be parenteral until observable clinical improvement is demonstrated, usually requiring 14 days of treatment.

Surgical intervention is not typically required except to preserve the function of the kidney or as a life-saving measure. Surgical intervention may become necessary to alleviate situations that lend themselves to recurrent infections and/or renal damage. These may include congenital anomalies, urogenital tract fistula, hypertrophic prostate, renal calculus (calculi), and vesicoureteral reflux. Surgical intervention may become emergent if the patient is febrile, has positive blood culture results for more than 48 hours, exhibits deterioration in condition, or appears toxic for more than 3 days (72 hours).

Complications

- Acute renal failure
- Chronic renal failure/damage
- Emphysematous cystitis
- Emphysematous pyelone-
  phritis
- Obstructing calculus
- Phrenic abscess
- Renal capillary necrosis
- Renal cortical abscess
  (renal carbuncle)
- Renal corticomedullary
  abscess
- Sepsis syndromes
- Staghorn calculus
- Xanthogranulomatous
  pyelonephritis

Anesthesia Implications

The nature or etiology of the patient's presentation to the operating room is an important factor for formulation of the anesthetic plan. The patient with pyelonephritis may present for emergent surgical intervention to rectify any of several conditions, such as emphysematous pyelonephritis or cystitis, phrenic abscess, or xanthogranulomatous pyelonephritis (see Complications above). The patient may be significantly febrile and dehydrated. Dehydration may result from the accompanying nausea and vomiting. Antibiotic therapy may be ongoing, and the anesthetist must be vigilant to adhere to the administration schedule for the antibiotics. Electrolyte imbalances, particularly potassium, are to be expected and may be partially the result of the significant emesis the patient may have. Both electrolyte concentrations and fluid balance should be determined preoperatively and corrective measures initiated as soon as possible. The patient may be septic, depending on the emergent condition precipitating the surgical intervention. The anesthetist should induce general anesthesia using the classic rapid sequence technique.

The anesthetist must ensure adequate intravenous access. Ideally, two large-bore IV catheters would be started before anesthesia to initiate adequate fluid resuscitation, maintain antibiotic administration schedule, and/or administer any vasopressors or vasoactive medications that may be required. Significantly febrile patients may require active cooling measures. The anesthetist may need to administer cooled IV fluid, apply cool packs to the axillae and/or groin, and use a forced-air cooling blanket to reduce the patient's temperature.

Frequently, the patient with pyelonephritis presenting emergently to the operating room requires complete or partial nephrectomy. As such, it may be necessary to place the patient in a lateral decubitus position. The anesthetist must take care

Factors Associated with Complicated Urinary Tract Infection

- Acquired immunodeficiency syndrome
- Acute renal colic
- Age over 65 years
- Analgesic abuse
- Bladder abscess
- Congenital immunodeficiency syndrome
- Diabetes mellitus
- Fistulae
- Foreign bodies (e.g., stents or calculi)
- Gross hematuria
- Hematogenous spread
- Infant/neonate
- Infected renal calculi
- Neurogenic bladder
- Neutropenia
- Nosocomial infection
- Obstruction
- Pregnancy
- Prior renal stones
- Renal impairment
- Renal transplant
- Resistant bacterial infection
- Sickle cell disease
- Tuberculosis
- Urinary diversion procedures
- Vesicoureteral reflux
- Yeast/fungal infection

P

to ensure proper positioning of the patient to prevent potential nerve injury. The anesthetist must also be acutely aware of the patient's respiratory status, especially the presence of any pulmonary co-morbidity factors that may be exacerbated by placing the patient in a lateral decubitus position. For example, pneumonia in a lobe of the dependent lung in the lateral position may reduce gas exchange and/or exacerbate any shunting that may be present.

P

> ## Recurrent Respiratory Papillomatosis

Definition

Recurrent respiratory papillomatosis (RRP) is a manifestation of infection by the human papilloma virus (HPV) anywhere within the entire respiratory tract/system, from the nose into the lungs.

Incidence

Age distribution of RRP is bimodal. The most common presentations are in children younger than 5 years, juvenile-onset recurrent respiratory papillomatosis (JORRP), or in adults in the fourth decade of life, known as adult-onset recurrent respiratory papillomatosis (AORRP). Children 14 years old or younger average 4.3 cases per 100,000 of the population. Adolescents 15 years to adult average 1.8 cases per 100,000 of the population.

In JORRP, males and females are affected equally. In AORRP, males are affected more frequently in a ratio approaching 4:1. RRP also seems to appear more frequently in Caucasians than other races.

Etiology

RRP is caused by the human papilloma virus (HPV), usually HPV-6 or HPV-11 variants. The HPV-16 or HPV-18 variants are the causative agents in rare cases.

JORRP is typically transmitted from the infected mother during the perinatal period, most commonly during vaginal delivery. JORRP produces a more severe disease than AORRP.

AORRP's mode of acquisition is not known with certainty, but it is strongly suspected to be via sexual transmission.

Signs and Symptoms

- Choking episodes
- Cough
- Dyspnea
- Failure to thrive
- Foreign body sensation
- Hoarseness
- Inspiratory wheeze
- Stridor
- Voice/vocal change
- Weak cry

R

Medical Management

Medical management of RRP consists almost entirely of surgical intervention. Pharmacotherapy is not a curative intervention but rather is intended to slow the growth of the HPV-produced papillomas and thereby extend the time between surgical debulking procedures. Pharmacologic agents with demonstrated effectiveness in increasing the intervals between resection or debulking include intralesional cidofovir, indole-3-carbinol, interferon, and photodynamic therapy. Other pharmacologic agents that have variable effects on RRP include cimetidine, acyclovir, and retinoic acid.

Curative intervention for RRP involves multiple surgical interventions (i.e., surgical debulking or resections). These procedures are performed with either the carbon dioxide laser, microdebridement, or cryotherapy. Frequently the resection is immediately followed by an injection into the resection site of cidofovir.

Microdebridement is preferred to laser debridement. The advantages of microdebridement include reductions in operative time, risk of infection for operating room personnel, and potential of airway burns. For laser resection, the carbon dioxide laser is preferred and affords better hemostasis during the operative procedure.

Photodynamic therapy has been the subject of small clinical trials. Results thus far show a reduced rate of papilloma formation. In this treatment method, dihematoporphyrin ether is administered 2 to 3 days before surgery. The therapy is accomplished by delivering an argon beam to the infected area either by laryngoscope or bronchoscope. The argon light activates the drug.

The airway of the patient with RRP should be repeatedly evaluated. For the newly diagnosed patient with RRP, the evaluations may be as frequent as every 2 to 4 weeks.

Complications

- Airway fire
- Airway/pulmonary burns
- Anterior glottic webbing or stenosis
- Negative-pressure pulmonary edema
- Pneumothorax
- Posterior glottic stenosis
- Solid or cystic pulmonary masses
- Subglottic edema
- Subglottic stenosis
- Tracheal stenosis

Anesthesia Implications

The first, and probably most critical, concern for the anesthetist caring for the patient with RRP revolves around securing the patient's airway. HPV papillomas in the respiratory tract may be found anywhere from the nose to, and into, the lungs. Most are found in the oropharynx, epiglottic, and glottic areas. With the patient awake, muscle tone may maintain an airway that is functionally adequate but quite tenuous. Induction of general anesthesia, with or without muscle paralysis, or even provision of a moderate degree of sedation may reduce the patient's muscle tone to the point of complete obstruction. The patient may become a "can't ventilate/can't intubate" patient almost instantly. Attempts at direct laryngoscopy must be undertaken with extreme caution; ideally, laryngoscopy should be delayed until the patient's airway reflexes are sufficiently suppressed, all the while striving to maintain spontaneous ventilations by the patient. Despite the apparent contradiction, this can be accomplished with a slow, careful, deliberate inhalation induction utilizing sevoflurane. If the patient is a small child, particularly one with stridor while at rest, the anesthetist should opt for an awake intubation. Intubation, whenever necessary, should be carried out with a smaller than usual endotracheal tube. Because of the high probability of papillomas in the oropharynx and the friability of those papillomas, the use of a laryngeal mask airway is best avoided.

Because of the close proximity of the surgical site to the patient's airway, whether natural or artificial, an airway fire is always a very real potential hazard. Airway fire can be particularly devastating and potentially fatal. The anesthetist must strive to use the lowest fraction of inspired oxygen possible, on the order of 0.25% to 0.35%, where feasible. The fraction of inspired oxygen should be reduced using helium (Helox) or nitrogen, but nitrous oxide should be avoided because it, too, supports combustion. The airway should be secured with either a special, laser-safe endotracheal tube or with an endotracheal tube wrapped with a reflective material, such as aluminum foil, to reduce the possibility of tube puncture and initiation of combustion. In the event of an airway fire, extinguishing it is the first priority. The steps to follow in the event of an airway fire are as follows: the endotracheal tube must be clamped, the balloon deflated, the tube removed, the patient ventilated by mask, and the airway inspected via direct laryngoscopy.

After these steps have been completed, the patient should be re-intubated if possible or the patient may require tracheostomy to secure the airway. The lower respiratory tract should be inspected via bronchoscopy and any visible debris removed, which may require bronchial lavage. The degree of pulmonary dysfunction produced by the thermal injury should be assessed by obtaining an arterial blood gas sample. The anesthetist may need to initiate supportive pharmacologic treatment in the form of corticosteroid(s) and antibiotics, plus racemic epinephrine combined with highly humidified oxygen. The surgical procedure will have to be terminated immediately with the exception of any necessary hemostasis.

Patients with RRP should remain intubated after the surgical procedure has been completed until their airway reflexes have fully returned, even in uncomplicated cases. The patient should not be extubated until fully awake because of the high potential for postoperative airway edema and compromise. For this same reason, the patient should receive humidified supplemental oxygen and be closely monitored postoperatively.

R

Sarcoidosis

Definition

Sarcoidosis is a chronic multisystem inflammatory disease characterized by noncaseating granulomas as well as lymphocytic alveolitis.

Incidence

In the United States the overall incidence of sarcoidosis ranges from 5:100,000 to 40:100,000. Among Caucasians the incidence is about 11:100,000, but among African Americans the incidence is about 34:100,000. Internationally the incidence varies with the country as well as the degree of development of the country. For example, in Sweden the incidence is about 20:100,000, whereas in Japan the incidence is about 1.3:100,000. Sarcoidosis has been reported in most countries. In developing countries it is frequently misdiagnosed as tuberculosis. This disease affects men more frequently than women by a 2:1 ratio.

Etiology

The true cause of sarcoidosis is not known. There is evidence of both genetic and environmental causative factors. Sarcoidosis is not a malignant disease, nor is it an autoimmune disease.

Possible Pathogenic Causes of Sarcoidosis
• Chlamydia
• Epstein-Barr virus
• Mycobacteria species
• Mycoplasma species

S

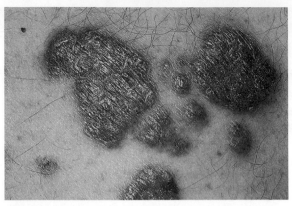

Sarcoidosis. Erythematous annular plaques. *(From Callen JP, et al:* Color Atlas of Dermatology, *ed 2, Philadelphia, 2000, Saunders.)*

Signs and Symptoms

- Alveolitis
- Anorexia
- Bell's palsy
- Deafness
- Depressed gag reflex
- Dysphagia
- Elevated monocyte count
- Fatigue
- Hepatomegaly
- Hilar lymphadenopathy
- Hoarseness
- Interstitial nephritis
- Iritis
- Night sweats
- Nonproductive cough
- Peripheral lymphade-
  nopathy
- Shortness of breath
- Skin lesions
- Splenomegaly
- T-cell lymphadenopathy
- Vertigo
- Vocal cord paralysis
- Weight loss

Medical Management

Symptomatic treatment is the only therapeutic measure most patients require. Corticosteroids currently remain the primary course of treatment, but noncorticosteroidal medications are increasingly being used. Methotrexate is often used in place of drugs such as prednisone. Other alternative medications include hydroxychloroquine, cyclosporine, pentoxifylline, and azathioprine. Sarcoidosis that proves refractory to any of these pharmacologic agents may be treated with infliximab and/or thalidomide. Cutaneous manifestations may be treated with tetracycline.

Pulmonary manifestations characterized by asymptomatic pulmonary function tests and/or chest x-rays may not require treatment. Symptomatic/abnormal pulmonary function test results and symptomatic chest x-ray findings generally signify that treatment is needed. Treatment is especially indicated with objective evidence of recent lung function deterioration. Administration of corticosteroids may produce some measure of improvement, but only a small degree. For endobronchial involvement, inhaled corticosteroids may be given.

Surgical intervention is limited. Bilateral lung transplantation is the most viable option for the patient with sarcoidosis in whom the disease has produced significant fibrosis. Transplantation is also an option for the sarcoidosis patient who is in Stage IV of the disease and should be seriously considered when the patient's forced vital capacity (FVC) and forced expiratory volume in 1 second (FEV_1) fall below 50% and 40%, respectively, of the patient's expected values.

Complications

- Cardiomyopathy
- Cor pulmonale
- Cranial nerve palsies
- Diabetes insipidus
- Encephalopathy
- End-stage lung disease
- Heart block
- Hypothalamic and/or pituitary dysfunction
- Lymphocytic meningitis
- Pericardial effusions
- Progressive pulmonary fibrosis
- Pulmonary hypertension
- Renal failure
- Right-side heart failure
- Seizures
- Sudden death

Anesthesia Implications

The first concern for the anesthetist whose patient has sarcoidosis centers on the degree of pulmonary involvement. Often there is significant disparity between expressed symptoms and the degree of pathologic changes. The patient's pulmonary function tests (PFTs) should be determined preoperatively, when possible. In addition, the patient's diffusing capacity and arterial blood gas analysis should be completed preoperatively to delineate the degree of hypoxemia and the impact the disease will have on the delivery of volatile anesthetics. Sarcoidosis produces significant loss of lung compliance, in this case producing restrictive lung disease. Both inspiratory and expiratory phases of the ventilation cycle should be prolonged to reduce the potential for barotrauma and air trapping. The inspiratory phase can be lengthened by selecting the pressure-controlled ventilation setting of most modern anesthesia machines along with lower peak inspiratory pressure settings for the inspiratory phase. The expiratory phase should be set for a ratio (I:E) of 1:2.5 or 1:3 to allow for more complete excursion. The loss of compliance along with decreased diffusing capacity produced by sarcoidosis may significantly alter the speed with which the depth of anesthesia can be changed. The anesthetist and the patient should have a preoperative discussion regarding the potential necessity of continuing mechanical ventilatory support into the postoperative period. Even when extubated, the patient must still be closely observed for a relatively longer time for signs of laryngeal edema and airway compromise, particularly for the patient with significant granulomatous infiltrates of the larynx. Patients with laryngeal involvement have been documented to suffer significant airway edema and compromise up to 36 hours postoperatively.

The second major concern for the anesthetist involves the degree of cardiac involvement. Cardiac involvement may be primary—directly the result of myocardial granuloma infiltration—or secondary—the result of the extensive pulmonary effects of the disease. Granulomatous infiltration of the myocardium may result in conduction abnormalities, such as first-degree atrioventricular conduction delay, bundle branch block, or even complete or third-degree heart block. It may also produce ventricular dysrhythmias, pericarditis, supraventricular tachycardia, ventricular aneurysms, or even sudden cardiac death. Myocardial effects of pulmonary manifestations may result in right-sided or congestive heart failure. The patient with sarcoidosis should have a 12-lead electrocardiograph evaluation performed preoperatively to detect any change in cardiac conduction abnormalities, along with a two-dimensional echocardiogram assessment to detect mechanical functional abnormalities resulting from the disease. Both studies should ideally be completed shortly before the anticipated surgery, preferably less than 30 days preoperatively, to alert the patient and anesthetist to any pathologic changes. The patient may require placement

S

of a pacemaker or internal cardiac defibrillator before the proposed surgical procedure, or the device may have already been implanted. Even though implanted for protective purposes, the internal defibrillator may have to be inactivated during surgery because the device may be triggered by electrocautery.

The patient with sarcoidosis may experience dysphagia and a depressed gag reflex as a result of granulomatous infiltration of cranial nerves (CN) IX and X, respectively. General anesthesia, when used, should be achieved via classic rapid sequence induction standards, with the patient's head elevated about 30 degrees to reduce the potential for aspiration. Extubation on completion of anesthesia requires that the patient be in very good control of his or her airway with return of protective reflexes. Humidified oxygen in the postoperative period will help soothe some of the airway irritation. The anesthetist must recall the greater potential for delayed airway compromise, particularly if the initial laryngoscopy and intubation were difficult to any degree. Signs and symptoms of laryngeal edema and/or airway compromise should be aggressively pursued and managed with dexamethasone and racemic epinephrine administration along with heightened observation and reintubation if necessary.

Intraoperatively, the patient with sarcoidosis may require placement of a pulmonary artery balloon floatation catheter and/or transesophageal cardiography probe to obtain more accurate data regarding fluid resuscitation and/or hemodynamic requirements. The patient may also benefit from placement of a peripheral arterial catheter for more accurate, beat-to-beat blood pressure monitoring, which will also facilitate serial arterial blood gas sampling perioperatively.

Cranial Nerve Effects of Sarcoidosis

Cranial Nerve	Effect
I	Olfactory problems
II	Visual disturbances
III, IV, VI	Ophthalmoplegia
VII	Bell's palsy/facial nerve paralysis
VIII	Deafness and vertigo
IX, X	Depressed gag reflexes, dysphagia
X	Hoarseness, vocal paralysis

S

The patient with sarcoidosis is typically treated with long-term corticosteroid administration. The anesthetist should take care to follow the established administration routine for perioperative steroid coverage.

Sarcoidosis may occasionally affect the kidneys. The anesthetist should be alert for the potential for renal insufficiency in the patient with sarcoidosis. The patient should have a complete metabolic panel obtained preoperatively to ascertain any electrolyte and/or fluid balance abnormalities.

Scleroderma

Definition

"Scleroderma" literally means "hard or thickened skin." The disease is a multisystem disorder characterized by inflammation, tissue fibrosis, and microvascular occlusion as the result of excessive production and deposition of collagen types I and III. Characteristics of scleroderma are most obvious in the skin but also appear in the pulmonary, cardiovascular, renal, gastrointestinal, and genitourinary systems.

Incidence

Scleroderma is found worldwide. Frequency is estimated at 19:1,000,000. Women have a 3- to 8-fold greater risk for developing the disease, with the peak onset between 30 and 50 years of age.

Etiology

The exact cause of scleroderma remains unknown. There are proposed pathologic mechanisms, such as endothelial cell injury, activation of fibroblasts, cytomegalovirus (human herpesvirus 5), and immune system derangement. Proposed environmental causative factors for scleroderma include exposure to silica or solvents such as trichloroethylene, epoxy resins, benzene, or carbon tetrachloride. To date, none of these proposed mechanisms have been substantiated.

Signs and Symptoms

- Arthralgia
- Aspiration pneumonia
- Bloating
- Chest pain
- Chronic renal insufficiency
- Constipation alternating with diarrhea
- Diffuse pruritus
- Dyspareunia
- Dyspepsia
- Dysphagia
- Early satiety
- Erectile dysfunction
- Facial pain
- Fatigue
- Gastroesophageal reflux
- Hand paresthesias
- Headache

S

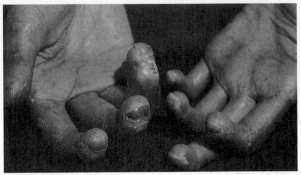

Scleroderma. Advanced systemic sclerosis. The extensive subcutaneous fibrosis has virtually immobilized the fingers, creating a clawlike flexion deformity. Loss of blood supply has led to cutaneous ulcerations. *(Courtesy of Richard Sontheimer, MD, Department of Dermatology, University of Texas Southwestern Medical School, Dallas, TX.)*

- Hoarseness
- Hyperpigmentation
- Hypopigmentation
- Hypothyroidism
- Incompetent lower esophageal sphincter
- Irregular heart rhythm
- Joint range of motion loss
- Muscle weakness
- Myalgia
- Palpitations
- Persistent dry cough
- Poor dentition
- Progressive dyspnea
- Pulmonary hypertension
- Raynaud phenomenon
- Renal crisis
- Sicca syndrome (see Sjögren syndrome, p. 316)
- Skin induration
- Skin tightness
- Stroke
- Syncope
- Weight loss

Medical Management

Currently, there is no FDA-approved treatment regimen specifically for scleroderma. Symptomatic or systematic treatments may be administered. No documented controlled studies have demonstrated a clear superiority of one treatment modality. The thickening of the patient's skin is frequently treated with D-penicillamine or methotrexate. Moisturizers, histamine-1 and -2 blocking drugs, tricyclic antidepressants, or trazodone may be used to treat the associated pruritus.

S

Raynaud phenomenon may be treated with calcium-channel blockers, prazosin, dipyridamole, aspirin, and/or topical nitrates. Tissue plasminogen activator, heparin, or urokinase may be needed in the event of thrombus formation and/or compromise of vascular flow.

Histamine-2 (H_2)-blockers, antacids, proton pump inhibitors, prokinetic medications, and/or octreotide may be used to treat the gastrointestinal manifestations of scleroderma. The patient may also need to exercise reflux precautions, consume smaller, more frequent meals, and/or laxatives to treat the gastrointestinal symptoms.

Pulmonary manifestations include fibrosis and hypertension. Cyclophosphamide, given either orally or intravenously, may be used to treat the patient's fibrosis. Pulmonary hypertension is initially treated with supplemental oxygen but may progress to the need for administration of bosentan in the most severe cases.

Corticosteroids, methotrexate, or azathioprine are generally used to treat the patient's myositis. Corticosteroids are usually the first line of drugs for this symptom. The dosage of steroids can be increased but only with great caution because doses greater than 40 mg/day can precipitate scleroderma-induced renal crisis. Every effort should be made to prevent initiation of a renal crisis associated with scleroderma, whether from the disease or from treatment of associated myositis. Angiotensin-converting enzyme inhibitor agents must be aggressively used with the first indication of the development of hypertension. Arthralgias and myalgias associated with scleroderma are usually treated with mild analgesics, such as acetaminophen and/or one of the nonsteroidal anti-inflammatory drugs.

Surgical intervention usually involves a digital sympathectomy. This relatively extreme intervention is generally reserved for those patients exhibiting a severe form of Raynaud phenomenon and who experience an acute, unrelenting episode that threatens one or more digits. Severely ischemic and/or infected digital lesions may necessitate debridement or, in the worst-case scenario, amputation. Severe flexion contractures may require surgical release.

Complications

- Cardiac tamponade
- Coagulation disorders
- Congestive heart failure
- Cor pulmonale
- Digital infarctions
- Infection
- Intestinal hypomotility
- Malabsorption syndrome
- Myositis
- Pericardial effusion
- Pericarditis
- Pulmonary fibrosis
- Pulmonary hypertension
- Renal failure
- Stroke

Anesthesia Implications

The first concern for the anesthetist is, as always, airway and breathing. Because of the relative tightness/tautness of the skin, the patient may have a limited range of motion of the mandible, thus poor opening of the mouth. It may therefore be difficult to perform direct laryngoscopy for intubation. The tightness is not affected by the administration of muscle relaxants. As a result, it may be necessary to secure the patient's airway via nasotracheal intubation, either blind or with the fiberoptic bronchoscope, or orally using the bronchoscope.

Skin manifestations of scleroderma are the most obvious, but pulmonary pathology from the disease is infinitely more complex and far reaching. Fibrotic pulmonary damage produces dramatic loss of lung compliance, resulting in restrictive pulmonary disease. The degree of the patient's restrictive disease should be determined preoperatively with pulmonary function tests (PFTs). In addition, the patient's lung function should be further evaluated by diffusion capacity testing and arterial blood gas sampling for analysis. The patient's fibrosis and altered lung compliance drastically increase the work of breathing. General anesthesia with preservation of spontaneous breathing is not recommended for the patient with scleroderma; therefore the employment of the laryngeal mask airway should be avoided. Mechanical ventilation of the patient may be difficult, requiring higher-than-expected pressure to inflate the lungs. Loss of compliance also means that expiration is generally not as complete as normal, making barotrauma a very real possibility. The anesthetist must attempt to provide mechanical ventilation with the lowest

S

possible peak inspiratory pressure while also providing a prolonged expiratory phase to reduce possible air trapping. Most of the more recent models of anesthesia machines allow for pressure-controlled ventilation, and the anesthetist should choose the lowest effective peak inspiratory pressure to provide good tidal volume and minute ventilation.

The patient with scleroderma should be evaluated for pulmonary hypertension by chest x-ray and electrocardiogram. Pulmonary hypertension heightens the patient's vulnerability to developing hypoxemia. Supplemental oxygen is of paramount importance for the patient no matter the scope of the proposed surgical intervention or the intended anesthesia technique. For the patient who will receive general anesthesia, the period of preoxygenation should extend beyond the recommended, typically 5 minutes, possibly even double that amount of time, assuming the procedure is not truly emergent in nature. Preoperative sedation should be maintained at a minimum, if given at all, and should definitely not incorporate opioid analgesics because of the patient's heightened vulnerability to develop hypoxemia. Intraoperatively, the anesthetist should not include nitrous oxide in the anesthetic plan because of the exacerbation of pulmonary hypertension that may result.

Before general anesthesia, the patient with scleroderma should receive pretreatment for gastroesophageal reflux using antacids and/or H_2-blockers to raise the pH of any gastric contents. Prokinetic agents may help promote gastric emptying before surgery and anesthesia. General anesthesia should be achieved via classic rapid sequence induction. At the end of anesthesia, the scleroderma patient should not be extubated until good laryngeal protective reflexes are demonstrated, whether in the operating room suite or in the post-anesthesia care unit.

Intravenous access may be difficult to obtain because of the toughness and thickness of the patient's skin. Intravenous access takes on a greater importance in the patient with scleroderma. The patient usually develops systemic hypertension as well as vasomotor instability. As a result, the patient adapts to life in a state of chronically reduced intravascular volumes, thus a state of relative hemoconcentration. When intravenous access is obtained, preferably via large-bore catheters, the anesthetist should "front-load" the patient with intravenous fluids in a fashion similar to the fluid loading given in preparation for

a regional anesthetic—providing the patient does not have
a history or symptoms of congestive heart failure. The fluid
load is intended to counteract the vasodilation produced by
induction of general anesthesia.

Regional anesthesia is an appropriate technique for the
patient with scleroderma, particularly those receiving total joint
arthroplasty procedures. Insertion of the needle for administration of the regional anesthetic may be difficult because of the
patient's thick skin, but also because of changes in joint mobility produced by the scleroderma. There have been reports
of prolonged action of local anesthetics in association with
scleroderma, but the etiology and/or clinical significance (if
any) have not been demonstrated.

Scleroderma can significantly alter kidney function and
result in renal failure. The functionality of the kidneys should
be assessed preoperatively. The anesthetist must temper anesthesia drug selection, as well as fluid resuscitation, in accor-
dance with the results of the renal function testing.

The patient with scleroderma may exhibit Raynaud phenomenon as well as sicca syndrome. Both must be accommo-
dated by the anesthetist. The Raynaud phenomenon should
be addressed by warming of the ambient room temperature to
about 70° F (21° C) administering warmed intravenous fluids,
and using a forced-air warming blanket throughout even the
shortest surgical procedure. Patients who exhibit a moderate to severe form of Raynaud phenomenon should not have
their radial artery catheterized for perioperative blood pressure
monitoring because of the heightened risk for digital ischemia.
Sicca syndrome causes excessive dryness of mucous membranes. As a result, antisialagogues should be omitted from the
patient's premedication orders. In addition, it is imperative that
the patient's eyes be lubricated and well protected throughout
the perioperative period.

Finally, malabsorption syndrome at times accompanies
scleroderma as the result of gastrointestinal manifestations of
the disease. Malabsorption can result in inadequate synthesis
of proteins, such as critical enzymes or clotting factors, or albumin.
Inadequate serum proteins can result in greater bioavailability
of some anesthesia medications, for which the anesthetist
may need to compensate by reducing the dose. In addition,

clotting factors may not be produced in appropriate concentrations, in which case the anesthetist should be prepared for greater than normal blood loss for a given surgical procedure. It may be appropriate to order blood typing and screening even for seemingly minor operative procedures, for which such blood work would not normally be necessary.

Shy-Drager Syndrome

Definition

Shy-Drager syndrome (SDS) is a sporadic, rare, progressive neurodegenerative disease characterized by features of parkinsonism, autonomic failure, and cerebellar or pyramidal dysfunction. Shy-Drager syndrome is also known as striatonigral degeneration, olivopontocerebellar atrophy, and multiple system atrophy.

Incidence

In the United States, the frequency of SDS is about 2:100,000 to 15:100,000. The frequency in other countries varies considerably. Men are more likely to be stricken than women, by a 3:1 to 9:1 ratio. Disease onset typically occurs between the ages of 52 and 55 years. The disease progresses over a period of 1 to 18 years, with a mean survival of 6 to 9.5 years.

Etiology

The cause of SDS is not known. There have been anecdotal suggestions of exposure to environmental toxins or trauma as causative agents, but none have been confirmed. Changes to the interomediolateral cell column have been documented as well as widespread brain anomalies. Neuronal losses have been documented in several brain regions.

Areas of Neuronal Loss in Shy-Drager Syndrome	
• Basal ganglia	• Pons
• Cerebellum	• Substantia nigra
• Hypothalamus	• Thalamus
• Locus ceruleus	• Vestibular complex
• Nucleus of Edinger-Westphal	

S

Signs and Symptoms

- Anhidrosis
- Ataxia
- Bowel dysfunction
- Bradykinesia
- Cardiac dysrhythmias
- Central sleep apnea
- Cerebellar uncoordination
- Chronic orthostatic hypotension
- Constipation
- Coarse leg tremors
- Dysdiadokinesia (inability to perform rapid, alternating movements)
- Dysmetria
- Episodic unconsciousness
- Erectile dysfunction
- Eye movement abnormalities
- Fasciculations
- Generalized neurologic dysfunction
- Muscle rigidity
- Muscle wasting
- Nausea
- Obstructive sleep apnea
- Paradoxical supine hypertension
- Truncal instability
- Urinary incontinence
- Vocal cord paralysis or dysfunction

Medical Management

There is no medical therapeutic measure, pharmacologic or nonpharmacologic, that can alter the course of Shy-Drager syndrome. It cannot be halted, reversed, or cured. Treatment measures are aimed at symptomatic relief. Orthostatic hypotension is a sentinel symptom for SDS patients and can dramatically interfere with a patient's daily life. Patients can incorporate various mechanical maneuvers to drastically reduce, if not alleviate, episodes of orthostatic hypotension (e.g., leg-crossing, squatting, abdominal compression, placing one foot on a chair). Paradoxical supine hypertension is a frequently occurring entity associated with SDS. To avoid the supine hypertension, patients are instructed not to lie down during the day. Sleeping at night with the head of the bed elevated about 30 degrees helps reduce the hypertension and the degree of orthostatic hypotension. There are several medications that may be used to treat orthostatic hypotension, such as fludrocortisone acetate, midodrine, dihydroxyphenylserine, epoetin alpha, indomethacin or ibuprofen, diphenhydramine, cimetidine, somastatin, octreotide, or desmopressin. The applicability of these pharmacologic interventions is limited by the supine hypertension. Patients who have profound bradycardia may have an atrial pacemaker inserted to treat the bradycardia and orthostatic hypotension.

S

The movement disorder of SDS may be treated with levodopa, dopaminergic agonists, anticholinergics, or amantadine. The response to these medications is usually favorable. The response produced is not as favorable, however, as that seen in patients with classic Parkinson's disease.

Complications

- Changes in alertness
- Delusions
- Disorientation
- Dizziness
- Hallucinations
- Injuries due to falls or syncope
- Involuntary movements
- Loss of mental function
- Nausea
- Progressive loss of ability to ambulate or care for self
- Severe confusion
- Side effects of medications for symptom alleviation
- Vomiting

Anesthesia Implications

Hemodynamic stability must be foremost in the mind of the anesthetist caring for the patient with SDS. The first step toward fostering the patient's hemodynamic stability should be to ensure optimization of the patient's fludrocortisone therapy. Perioperatively the patient should be invasively monitored with interarterial cannulization as well as central venous pressure and/or pulmonary artery catheterization, depending on the complexity of the intended surgery, to guide fluid resuscitation and blood loss replacement. Crystalloids, colloids (fluid expanders), and blood or blood products should be given to preserve normotension by maintaining normovolemia because the patient's response to vasoactive amines is unpredictable. The autonomic denervation that occurs with this disease process produces sympathetic hypersensitivity. As a result, vasoactive amines must be administered judiciously to treat intraoperative hypotension using significantly reduced doses.

Supine hypertension, which is common with this disease, has been treated with labetalol, but the response reported was minimal. However, administration of hydralazine to treat supine hypertension produced a profound hypotension that could only be rectified with a vasopressin infusion. The supine hypertension does respond quite favorably to either a sodium nitroprusside infusion or transdermal nitroglycerin application.

S

Regional anesthesia is effective in patients with SDS. Patients with SDS tolerate the regional anesthesia–induced sympathectomy considerably better (i.e., without the hypotension generally observed) than unaffected patients, possibly because they are already experiencing a constant sympathectomy as a result of the disease process.

General anesthesia can be achieved and maintained with any of the volatile agents. There have been no reports of unexpected untoward effects from any of the currently available anesthetic agents. The anesthetist should keep in mind that central sleep apnea, obstructive sleep apnea, and stridor are all commonly seen in patients with SDS. Prior planning, understanding, and cooperation with the patient are required with regard to extubation at the end of surgery, particularly for a patient with a history of either form of sleep apnea or with a history of stridor. The anesthetist may wish to somewhat reduce the dose of benzodiazepine and/or opioid because of the heightened potential for respiratory embarrassment. It may be prudent to arrange for an overnight observation in the intensive care unit so that the patient's respiratory status can be closely monitored for the first 24 hours postoperatively.

Sjögren Syndrome

Definition

Sjögren syndrome is a complex disorder in which exocrine organs are infiltrated by lymphocytes. It is characterized by sicca symptoms and is frequently associated with systemic lupus erythematosus, rheumatoid arthritis, or scleroderma.

Incidence

The estimated incidence of Sjögren syndrome is 0.1% to 3%; the wide estimated range is due to the lack of uniform diagnostic criteria. Females are affected more often than males by a 9:1 ratio.

Etiology

The etiology of Sjögren syndrome is not truly known. Theoretically there appear to be interactions between major histocompatibility complex (MHC) genetic factors and non-MHC genetic factors, along with still-undelineated environmental factors. Sex hormones are theorized to play a role because of the overwhelming tendency of this disease to affect women.

Signs and Symptoms

Sicca Symptoms
- Parotid enlargement
- Xerophthalmia
- Xerostomia
- Xerotrachea

Other
- Anemia
- Arthralgia
- Arthritis
- Dementia
- Fatigue
- Gastrointestinal disease
- Interstitial lung disease
- Leukopenia
- Lymphadenopathy
- Lymphoma

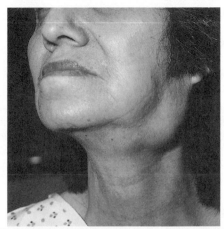

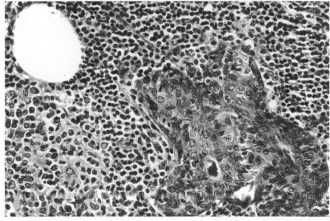

Sjögren Syndrome. Enlargement of the salivary gland. *(Courtesy of Richard Sontheimer, MD, Department of Dermatology, University of Texas Southwestern Medical School, Dallas, TX.)*

S

- Myalgia
- Neuropathy
- Palpable purpura
- Pneumonitis
- Pulmonary disease

- Raynaud phenomenon
- Recurrent bronchitis
- Renal tubular acidosis
- Seizures
- Vasculitis

Medical Management

Treatment interventions for the patient with Sjögren syndrome are dictated by the symptoms the patient experiences. Sicca symptoms are treated by moisturizing interventions (e.g., xerophthalmia is treated with artificial tears; xerostomia is treated with liberal sips of water or sugar-free lemon drops to stimulate saliva production). More detailed interventions may be required that are dictated by the presence of an associated rheumatic disease such as systemic lupus erythematosus (see p. 335), rheumatoid arthritis, or scleroderma (see p. 305).

Complications

- Antiphospholipid syndrome
- Emergence of pseudolymphomas
- Emergence of systemic lupus erythematosus, rheumatoid arthritis, or scleroderma
- Parotid gland infection
- Parotid gland tumor

Anesthesia Implications

The anesthetist should continue interventions aimed at alleviation of sicca symptoms. The patient is particularly prone to corneal injury. Instilling eye lubricant and taping the eyelids closed during anesthesia are imperative for the patient with Sjögren syndrome. It is appropriate for the anesthetist to swab the patient's mouth with some type of moisturizer perioperatively. To combat the patient's xerotrachea, the anesthetist should use warmed, humidified gases throughout the duration of the anesthetic, whether general anesthesia, regional anesthesia, or monitored anesthesia care.

S

The anesthetist should anticipate that the patient with Sjögren syndrome may present with a difficult airway. Mask fit may be difficult to obtain because of enlargement of submandibular and/or parotid glands. Enlargement of these glands may hinder the anesthetist's ability to visualize the patient's vocal cords to intubate the patient. For more specific information regarding anesthesia implications, refer to the discussions of rheumatoid arthritis, systemic lupus erythematosus (p. 335), and scleroderma (p. 305).

Stevens-Johnson Syndrome

Definition

Stevens-Johnson syndrome (SJS) is a hypersensitivity disorder mediated by immune-complex formation. It is a potentially fatal systemic disorder that is a severe type of erythema multiforme. SJS is also known as "erythema multiforme major."

Incidence

The frequency of SJS is estimated to be about 1.2:1,000,000 to 6:1,000,000. This disorder has been reported in all racial and ethnic groups and affects both sexes about equally over all age groups.

Etiology

Stevens-Johnson syndrome is classified into four categories (see box below). Approximately half of all cases of SJS have been linked to ingestion of a medication. To date, more than 100 different medications have been linked to the development of SJS (see box on pp. 321-322). The second most common cause result from infectious agents/vectors (see box on p. 321). As many as 25% of SJS cases are deemed idiopathic, while the smallest number of SJS cases have been associated with some form of carcinoma and/or lymphoma.

Four Etiologic Categories of Stevens-Johnson Syndrome
1. Infectious
2. Drug-induced
3. Malignancy-related
4. Idiopathic

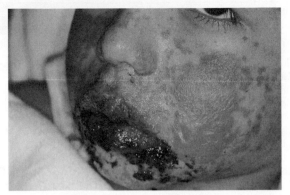

Stevens-Johnson Syndrome. Severe oral and skin involvement. *(From Weston WL, Lane AT, Morelli JB:* Color Textbook of Pediatric Dermatology, *ed. 4, St. Louis, 2007, Mosby.)*

Infectious Causes of Stevens-Johnson Syndrome

- Adenoviruses
- Calmette-Guérin virus
- Deep fungal infections
- Enterobacter species
- Enteroviruses
- Herpes simplex virus
- Influenza
- Measles
- Mumps
- *Mycobacterium pneumoniae*
- *Mycobacterium tuberculosis*
- *Streptococcus pneumoniae*
- Syphilis
- Typhoid fever

Drugs Associated with the Development of Stevens-Johnson Syndrome

Sulfonamides
- Pyrimethamine-sulfadoxine (Fansidar)
- Sulfadiazine (Coptin)
- Sulfasalazine (Azulfidine)
- Trimethoprim-sulfamethoxazole

Anticonvulsants
- Carbamazepine
- Phenobarbital
- Phenytoin (Dilantin)

Others
- Acetaminophen
- Allopurinol (Aloprim, Zyloprim)
- Aminopenicillins
- Amithiozone
- Amoxapine (Asendin)
- Barbiturates
- Cephalosporins
- Chlormezanone (Trancopal)
- Clobazam

Continued

S

Drugs Associated with the Development of Stevens-Johnson Syndrome—cont'd

- Diclofenac
- Fluvoxamine (Luvox)
- Hydantoins
- Imidazole antifungals
- Indapamide (Lozol)
- Lamotrigine (Lamictal)
- Macrolides
- Mianserin
- Oxicam
- Nonsteroidal anti-inflammatory drugs (NSAIDs) (piroxicam, tenoxicam)
- Propionic NSAIDs
- Propranolol (Inderal, InnoPran XL)
- Pyrazolone derivatives (i.e., dipyrone)
- Quinolones
- Salicylates
- Sertraline (Zoloft)
- Tetracycline
- Tiapride
- Trazodone
- Valproic acid (Depakene, myproic acid)

Signs and Symptoms

- Altered level of consciousness
- Anxiety
- Arthralgia
- Coma
- Confluent erythema
- Conjunctivitis
- Corneal ulcerations
- Dehydration
- Dysuria
- Epistaxis
- Erosive vulvovaginitis
- Fever
- Headache
- Hyperventilation
- Hypotension
- Malaise
- Mild hypoxia
- Mucous membrane erythema, edema, sloughing, blisters, ulceration, and/or necrosis
- Mucous membrane lesions (e.g., oropharynx, conjunctivae, genitalia, anus, tracheobronchial tree, esophagus, bowel)
- Orthostasis
- Productive cough (thick and purulent)
- Profuse diarrhea
- Purpuric macules, papules, vesicles, or bullae
- Seizures
- Tachycardia
- Urticarial plaques

Medical Management

The most critical step is early detection of SJS followed by rapid, aggressive initiation of treatment. The patient begins treatment by discontinuing use of any medications that may be the potential causative agent. The disorder causes significant disruption of the patient's skin barrier that closely resembles the denuded appearance of chemical or thermal burn injuries. This disorder is essentially a "burn" produced by internal mechanisms that disrupt skin and/or mucous membrane integrity—almost as if the patient is "burned" from the inside outward. The patient also frequently experiences profuse diarrhea along with significant increases in core temperature.

These symptoms—skin loss, diarrhea, and hyperthermia—may cause the patient to lose significant fluid volume. Fluid losses frequently bring about extensive shifts/losses of electrolyte concentrations. The fluid volume losses must be aggressively treated to avoid potentially lethal losses culminating in cardiovascular collapse. Fluid resuscitation requirements are generally 66% to 75% of the amount necessary to care for a burn-injured patient with a comparably sized injury. Fluid should be given via peripheral intravenous access that is as distant from the cutaneous or mucosal lesions and/or denuded areas as possible. Resuscitation via central venous access should be avoided if at all possible because of a greater potential for infection. Fluids should be warmed (if the patient is not significantly febrile) to prevent initiation of shivering, which can increase oxygen consumption by as much as 300%.

There is no single medication that can successfully treat SJS. The preponderance of treatments address symptoms. Denuded skin areas are generally treated with bactericidal creams. Occasionally, surgical intervention may be required to promote skin regeneration by application of xenographs and similar interventions.

If the tracheobronchial tree is involved, it will be manifested by hyperventilation plus mild hypoxemia. Aggressive pulmonary support is required to detect the onset of diffuse interstitial pneumonitis. With early detection of the pneumonitis, treatment can be initiated sooner to reduce the potential for, if not prevent, acute respiratory distress syndrome (ARDS).

Similar to the treatment of burn injuries, pain control is a significant problem. The skin disruption of SJS is strikingly similar to that of a deep partial-thickness thermal or chemical injury; the nerve endings are basically uncovered and are constantly in a state of hyperstimulation. Attaining adequate analgesia may require potent opioid analgesics. In addition, the patient with SJS is prone to develop stress ulcers. The patient should be treated with antacids, histamine-2 (H_2)-blockers, and/or proton pump inhibitors. The patient should be placed on deep vein thrombosis prophylaxis, which may include use of heparin.

SCORTEN Score Prognostic Factors and Mortality Rates

Variables
- Age >40 years
- Bicarbonate <20 mmol/L
- BUN >10 mmol/L
- Heart rate >120 bpm
- Initial percentage of epidermal detachment >10%
- Malignancy
- Serum glucose >14 mmol/L

Scores and Mortality Rates

Score	Mortality Rate
0-1	≥3.2%
2	≥12.1%
3	≥35.3%
4	≥58.3%
5	≥90%

Complications

- ARDS
- Blindness
- Burning eyes
- Conjunctival synechiae
- Corneal and conjunctival neovascularization
- Corneal scarring
- Death
- Epithelial proliferation with squamous metaplasia
- Esophageal strictures
- In-turned eyelashes
- Lacrimal duct obstruction causing epiphora
- Nephritis
- Patchwork skin
- Penile scarring
- Photophobia
- Pneumonia
- Renal tubular necrosis
- Sjögren-like sicca syndrome (see p. 316)
- Tracheobronchial shedding with respiratory failure
- Vaginal synechiae
- Visual impairment

Anesthesia Implications

The skin of the patient with SJS is extremely fragile; lesions may develop easily and just as easily rupture to produce a new skin barrier disruption. Anesthetists must take extraordinary care when positioning the patient and padding bony prominences and pressure points. The best padding for the patient with SJS is to use gelatin-filled pads that

S

maximize the dispersal of pressure. In addition, the patient with SJS should have his or her skin protected from the shearing forces the blood pressure cuff can produce, which will exacerbate skin barrier disruption. Similarly, securing intravenous catheters, endotracheal tubes, and protecting the eyes with tape can be detrimental to the patient with SJS because removal of the tape can also remove the underlying skin. Intravenous lines may be best secured using a suture rather than tape, followed by covering the site with a sterile gauze dressing. The endotracheal tube can be secured using any of the commercially available devices. The patient's eyes can be protected by placing lightly moistened gauze pads on the closed eyes then wrapping the head with gauze. The anesthetist should also take similar care when removing the electrocardiogram pads and should strive to minimize the shearing forces produced.

Intravenous access is a critical need for the patient with SJS for both anesthesia administration and fluid resuscitation. Central venous access is discouraged. However, if larger fluid volumes are required, it is obviously an avenue to be cautiously explored after weighing the risks versus benefits. The patient will have nutritional needs similar to those of a patient with burn injuries and may need to receive parenteral nutrition on arrival at the operating room. It is important that the parenteral nutrition be maintained throughout the duration of the anesthetic. The patient also may be receiving enteral nutritional support critical to the healing process. Although it presents the risks of a full stomach, the anesthetist should allow the supplementation to continue, possibly at a slower rate, until the patient is delivered to the operating room to be prepared for anesthesia. Induction of general anesthesia must, of necessity, follow the classic rapid sequence induction precautions.

The patient with SJS frequently has significant involvement of the oral cavity and oropharynx, and may present with major laryngeal edema. These tissues will be almost astoundingly friable. Hemorrhagic bullae form with seemingly the most simple contact; direct laryngoscopy, endotracheal intubation, oral and nasal airway insertion, placement of an esophageal stethoscope, or passing an orogastric or nasogastric tube may produce and rupture these bullae and cause immediate severe airway compromise. The use of a laryngeal mask airway is not strictly contraindicated in the patient with SJS, but its use must be very carefully considered, especially in the patient with extensive oral cavity involvement, despite the reduced use of positive pressure ventilation it can afford.

The involvement of mucous membranes in the patient with SJS can extend further down the tracheobronchial tree, resulting in development of visceral pleural blebs. These blebs are likely to rupture, producing pneumothorax. For this reason it is desirable to avoid positive pressure ventilation where possible. In cases where positive pressure ventilation is unavoidable, it is advisable to prolong the inspiratory phase with reduced peak inspiratory pressure by selecting a pressure-controlled method of ventilation available on most late-model anesthesia machines. At the same time, the lowest effect peak inspiratory pressure should be selected as well. These measures will help minimize the potential for bleb rupture. In addition, because of its rapid diffusion and expansion, nitrous oxide should not be used, especially if tracheobronchial tree involvement and/or pleural bleb formation is suspected.

Because of the patient's high degree of pain, potent opioid analgesics may be in use with adequate or inadequate pain relief. The anesthetist should anticipate that the patient has developed tolerance to the opioid analgesics and should be prepared to administer large doses of opioids to achieve seemingly minimal results. No specific anesthesia drugs or anesthesia techniques have demonstrated clear superiority for the patient with SJS. Infiltration of local anesthetic must be undertaken cautiously, with due consideration for the condition of the patient's skin as well as the increased potential for infection. Drugs that have been implicated in the development of SJS, such as barbiturates, should be avoided. Propofol has been used safely to anesthetize patients with SJS, as has ketamine. Both can be used as the sole anesthetic agent if necessary. The anesthetist must also consider the route of elimination for anesthesia-related drugs when planning the anesthesia care for the patient with SJS. In particular, the anesthetist should avoid potentially nephrotoxic drugs and those eliminated via the kidneys when renal involvement has been demonstrated.

Sturge-Weber Syndrome

Definition

Sturge-Weber syndrome (SWS) is a congenital disorder characterized by leptomeningeal angiomas as well as cutaneous angiomas along distributions of the trigeminal nerve (usually only on one side), in particular the ophthalmic and maxillary tracts. The cutaneous angioma is known as the port-wine stain or port-wine angioma. Sturge-Weber syndrome is also called encephalotrigeminal angiomatosis and Sturge-Kalischer-Weber syndrome.

Roach Scale Classification of Sturge-Weber Syndrome	
Type I	Facial and leptomeningeal angiomas; may have glaucoma
Type I	Facial angioma only; may have glaucoma
Type III	Isolated leptomeningeal angioma; usually does not have glaucoma

Incidence

The incidence of SWS is estimated to be 1:50,000.

Etiology

The etiology of SWS is not clear. The angiomas appear to develop as the result of a somatic mutation that alters the structure, function, and innervation of blood vessels, expressed as seen in the extracellular matrix and vasoactive molecules. SWS is seen in people of all races and both genders.

Signs and Symptoms

- Attention deficit hyperactivity disorder
- Buphthalmos (congenital glaucoma)
- Choroidal angioma
- Glaucoma
- Headache
- Hemianopsia
- Hemiparesis
- Heterochromia of the iris
- Macrocephaly
- Mental retardation

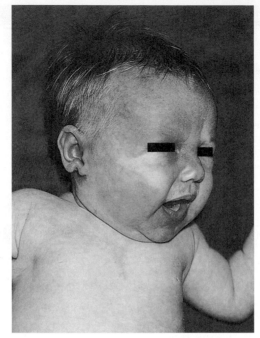

Sturge-Weber Syndrome. Port wine stain on infant who subsequently developed seizures with Sturge-Weber syndrome. *(From Weston WL, Lane AT, Morelli JG: Color Textbook of Pediatric Dermatology, ed. 4, St Louis, 2007, Mosby.)*

- Port wine stain or angioma
- Seizures
- Soft-tissue hypertrophy
- Stroke
- Tomato-catsup colored fundus of the eye
- Vision loss
- Weakness

Medical Management

The primary medical concerns for care of the patient with SWS include seizure control, headache relief (both symptomatic and prophylactic), reduction of intraocular pressure, and removal of the port-wine stain. Seizure control is typically achieved with administration of anticonvulsant medications. Seizures associated with SWS are generally focal and, as a result, frequently respond well to anticonvulsant therapy.

Gaining control of the patient's intraocular pressure is achieved with standard glaucoma medications used to lower the intraocular pressure either by reducing aqueous fluid production or by enhancing/promoting the outflow of aqueous fluid.

Headaches are generally recurrent and are treated with acetaminophen or ibuprofen for analgesia. Prophylactic measures may include more proactive/preventive medications, such as gabapentin, valproate, or amitriptyline. Stroke-like episodes may be treated with aspirin in doses from 3 to 5 mg/kg/day. However, because of the risk for Reye syndrome, aspirin use in children must be undertaken with caution.

Port-wine stain is evident at birth and must be closely evaluated within the first week of life, as well as differentiated from hemangioma. Treatment of port-wine stain is accomplished with laser therapy. The number of laser treatments required depends on the extensiveness of the area affected by the port-wine stain. The treatments should be initiated as soon as possible.

Surgical intervention for the patient with SWS is generally reserved for those with refractory seizures, unresponsive or poorly controlled glaucoma, or for specific problems (most notably, scoliosis). In some instances, the seizures of a patient with SWS become refractory to pharmacologic interventions, and the patient may deteriorate to a state of status epilepticus. Surgical interventions for medically refractory seizures include focal cortical resection, corpuscallosotomy, vagal nerve stimulation, and hemispherectomy. Some investigators advocate early surgical intervention to prevent refractory seizures, developmental delay, or hemiparesis. Others advocate exploratory craniotomy and possible lobectomy on confirmation of the diagnosis of SWS because of evidence that links early-onset seizures with developmental delay and/or mental retardation.

Cranial Surgery Indications in Sturge-Weber Syndrome

- Cognitive function deterioration
- Early (age) onset of seizures
- Extensive leptomeningeal angioma
- Focal seizures, subsequently generalized
- Headaches/mild trauma associated with transient motor deficits
- Hemiparesis development
- Increasing duration of postictal deficit
- Increasing focal or diffuse atrophy
- Increasing frequency and duration of seizures
- Medically refractory seizures
- Permanent motor deficits
- Progressive atrophy or calcifications
- Progressive neurologic damage

Indications of Sturge-Weber Syndrome Progression

- Deterioration of cognitive function
- Development of hemiparesis
- Focal seizures initially progress in frequency, secondarily to general, seizures
- Increased duration of transient postictal deficits
- Increased focal or diffuse atrophy
- Increased frequency of seizures (initially) despite anticonvulsant/ antiepileptic drugs
- Increased progression of calcifications

When pharmacologic therapy is unsuccessful in controlling intraocular pressure, surgical intervention may be necessary. Trabeculectomy promotes the outflow of aqueous fluid from the anterior chamber by reopening the anatomical outflow tract. Goniotomy accomplishes the same goal intraocularly rather than extraocularly. A Molteno valve, which is analogous to a shunt, may be inserted to promote outflow of anterior chamber aqueous fluid, while the production of aqueous fluid may be reduced by employing cyclodestructive procedures that use cryogenic applications or laser treatments.

Complications

- Blindness
- Buphthalmos (congenital glaucoma)
- Cognitive dysfunction deterioration
- Glaucoma
- Hemianopsia
- Hemiparesis
- Hydrocephalus
- Increased intracranial pressure
- Refractory seizures
- Status epilepticus
- Stroke

Anesthesia Implications

The patient with SWS most often presents to the operating room for treatment of the port-wine stain, refractory seizures, uncontrolled glaucoma, or ocular angioma. The patient should be evaluated preoperatively for untoward intracranial developments, such as increased intracranial pressure (ICP) and/or hydrocephalus. Further evaluation is required with regard to the patient's potential neurologic pathology and delineation of any associated symptoms. If the surgery is not directed toward regaining control of seizure activity or eliminating seizures,

S

the patient's anticonvulsant therapy should be optimized before surgery whenever possible.

The patient presenting with signs and symptoms of hydrocephalus and/or ICP should be hyperventilated to begin reducing the diameter of cerebral blood vessels, thus reducing the intracranial pressure. Additional measures to help "relax" the brain include inducing diuresis with an osmotic agent, such as mannitol, and use of sufentanil for analgesia.

The anesthetist must keep in mind the close association of glaucoma with SWS. Topical β-blocking agents used to decrease intraocular pressure can produce systemic effects, including bradycardia and asthma exacerbation. Cholinesterase inhibitors (echothiophate) may decrease plasma cholinesterase, thus prolonging the effects of succinylcholine. Long-term use of acetazolamide may result in sodium and bicarbonate diuresis as well as metabolic acidosis. Where possible, glaucoma medications should be continued perioperatively, with the exception of echothiophate, which should be discontinued 2 to 3 weeks before surgery. Discontinuation of echothiophate can result in exacerbation of glaucoma. The anesthetist should avoid succinylcholine in the patient with SWS, whether echothiophate has been discontinued or not, because of its tendency to elevate intraocular pressure.

The patient with SWS, particularly one being treated with acetazolamide, should have a basic metabolic panel completed preoperatively to assess the sodium concentration and determine the possible need for arterial blood gas analysis to measure the bicarbonate concentration. Direct laryngoscopy for intubation should be accomplished as quickly as possible because of the associated elevation in intraocular pressure. Laryngeal mask airway use does not produce such intraocular pressure elevation and may be a good choice for appropriate surgical procedures. The anesthetist may wish to consider extubation while the patient is relatively deeply anesthetized (so-called "deep extubation") to minimize the coughing, straining, and/or bucking on the endotracheal tube, which, in turn, elevates the intraocular pressure.

Sydenham's Chorea

Definition

Sydenham's chorea (SC) is a self-limiting disorder most often seen in children from 5 to 15 years of age. It may also manifest during pregnancy. This disease is often linked with rheumatic fever and is marked by involuntary movements that can become severe enough over time to affect all motor activities. Sydenham's chorea is also known as St. Vitus' dance and rheumatic chorea.

Incidence

The frequency of SC is related to the incidence of rheumatic fever. SC is estimated to occur in 10% to 20% of patients with rheumatic fever. In the United States, the incidence of rheumatic fever is 0.5:100,000 to 2:100,000. The incidence of SC would be estimated to be about 0.05:100,000 to 0.4:100,000. Internationally, the incidence of rheumatic fever is much higher in developing and underdeveloped countries where antibiotic treatments are much less available. Therefore the incidence of SC is higher in these countries.

Etiology

The underlying cause of SC is infection by the Lancefield group A β-hemolytic streptococcal organism, which apparently contributes to the development of antineuronal antibodies. The antineuronal antibodies cross-react with an unknown epitope in basal ganglia neurons.

Signs and Symptoms

- Deterioration of hand writing
- Emotional lability
- Facial grimacing
- Hypotonia
- Involuntary movements
- Irritability
- Muscle weakness
- Restlessness
- Slow or slurred speech

Medical Management

Sydenham's chorea is usually a self-limiting disorder.
The patient typically "outgrows" the disorder. Treatment
is generally reserved for patients in whom the chorea
becomes severe enough to interfere with daily functioning.
Choreiform movements may be controlled with valproic
acid; improvement is usually seen within 7 days of treatment
initiation. Carbamazepine, an anticonvulsant, and diazepam
may also produce desired results. Choreiform movements
can also be controlled using dopaminergic blockers and
depletors; however, their use has been constrained by the
significant side effects they are known to produce.

Complications

- Cardiac conduction defects secondary to rheumatic fever
- Choreoathetosis
- Endocarditis
- Relapse of streptococcal infection
- Rheumatism

Anesthesia Implications

The close association of SC with a history of rheumatic
fever should cause the anesthetist to focus on cardiac
abnormalities that may have been produced by the streptococcal infection. The patient should receive a thorough
preoperative cardiac evaluation, including a 12-lead
electrocardiogram, even though the patient is younger than
20 years of age.

The patient should also receive prophylactic antibiotic
coverage as a preventive measure related to the history of
β-hemolytic streptococcal infection and rheumatic fever. The
patient's medication profile or history should be reviewed.
The patient with SC may be undergoing treatment with corticosteroids, barbiturates, phenothiazines, and/or antiparkinsonian
medications such as levodopa. Perioperative continuation
of corticosteroids is particularly important because of the
possible adrenal suppression long-term corticosteroid use
can produce.

Administration of anesthesia to a patient with SC has
been a rare event. Because anesthetic experience with SC

S

patients is so limited, no technique or agent has been
specifically recommended or contraindicated. The primary
anesthetic concerns involve potential drug interactions
from medications being used for the patient's symptomatic
treatment.

Systemic Lupus Erythematosus

Definition

Systemic lupus erythematosus (SLE) is a chronic, generalized, multifaceted inflammatory disorder that can affect every organ. SLE is categorized as an autoimmune disease characterized by autoantibody formation, producing multisystem microvascular inflammation.

Incidence

In the United States the average incidence of SLE is about 1:10,000. The incidence varies with ethnicity. The female: male ratio ranges from 8:1 to 10:1. Internationally the incidence is variable by country and ethnicity (see the table below).

Prevalence Variations	
Country	Frequency
Great Britain	12:100,000
Sweden	39:100,000
New Zealand/Polynesian heritage	50:100,000
New Zealand/Caucasian	14.6:100,000

Etiology

The specific cause of SLE has not yet been elucidated. There are suspected causes, including immune system dysregulation as well as immune complex tissue damage—particularly in the skin and kidneys. Development of SLE may result from multiple immune disturbances. In addition, 10 gene loci have been implicated in increased risk of development of SLE.

S

American College of Rheumatology Systemic Lupus Erythematosus Diagnosis Criteria

This is called the SOAP BRAIN MD mnemonic:

Serositosis	Pleurisy, pericarditis
Oral ulcers	Oral or nasopharyngeal, usually painless; the palate is most specific
Arthritis	Nonerosive, Jaccoud-type
Photosensitivity	Unusual skin reaction to light exposure
Blood disorders	Leukopenia, lymphopenia, thrombocytopenia, positive result of Coombs-test for anemia
Renal involvement	Proteinuria (>0.5 g/day)
Antinuclear antibodies (ANAs)	Higher titers generally more specific (>1:160)
Immunologic phenomena	Lupus erythematosus (LE) cells; anti–double-stranded DNA (dsDNA); anti-Smith (Sm) antibodies; antiphospholipid antibodies; lupus; anticoagulants
Neurologic disorder	Seizures or psychosis
Malar rash	Fixed erythema over the cheeks and nasal bridge
Discoid rash	Raised rimmed lesions that have keratotic scaling and follicular plugging

Signs and Symptoms

- Alopecia
- Anasarca
- Aseptic meningitis
- Bullous lesions
- Crackles
- Diffuse intrapulmonary hemorrhage
- Dysrhythmias
- Effusions
- Fever
- Fibromyalgia
- Focal neurologic deficits
- Gross hemoptysis
- Heart failure
- Hematuria
- Hypertension
- Hypoxia
- Infectious endocarditis
- Inflammatory myocarditis
- Ischemia
- Jaccoud arthropathy/arthritis/syndrome
- Libman-Sacks disease (atypical verrucous endocarditis)
- Lymphadenopathy
- Malar rash
- Mesenteric vasculitis
- Mononeuritis
- Myositis
- Oral ulcers
- Organic brain syndrome (currently defined as delirium, dementia,

S

and amnestic and other cognitive disorders; mental disorder from general medical condition; and substance-related disorder)
- Palatal ulcers
- Pancreatitis
- Panniculitis
- Periorbital edema
- Peripheral edema
- Peritonitis
- Photosensitive rash
- Plaque-like lesions with follicular plugging
- Pleuropericardial friction rubs
- Pneumonitis
- Psychosis
- Pulmonary embolism
- Raynaud phenomenon
- Seizures
- Splenomegaly
- Tachypnea
- Urticaria
- Vasculitic purpura

Medical Management

Treatment of SLE is not curative; rather, it addresses symptoms. Treatment plans are developed based on the patient's age, sex, health status, symptoms, and lifestyle. Changes in the patient's symptom profile over time require changes or alterations in the treatment regimen. The goals of SLE treatment are to produce symptomatic relief, prevent exacerbations of the disease, treat the exacerbations when they occur, and minimize organ damage and complications. Pharmacologic agents used in SLE treatment regimens include nonsteroidal anti-inflammatory drugs (NSAIDs), antimalarials, corticosteroids, and immune suppressants.

Complications

- Anemia
- Behavioral changes
- Endocarditis
- Kidney damage
- Myocardial infarction
- Myocarditis
- Opportunistic infection(s)
- Osteonecrosis
- Pericarditis
- Pleurisy
- Premature atherosclerotic heart disease
- Renal failure
- Seizures
- Vasculitis

Anesthesia Implications

Preoperative concerns for the patient with SLE center primarily on the renal and pulmonary manifestations of the disease. Secondary concerns center on any cardiac manifestations.

Pulmonary Manifestations

- Bronchiolitis
- Chronic interstitial lung disease
- Diffuse alveolar hemorrhage
- Interstitial pneumonia
- Lupus pleuritis

- Lupus pneumonitis
- Pulmonary embolism
- Pulmonary hypertension
- Respiratory muscle dysfunction

Preoperatively, the patient with SLE should have serum creatinine and blood urea nitrogen (BUN) levels determined to ascertain the degree of renal involvement. The anesthetist must take care to avoid drugs heavily dependent on renal excretion if renal insufficiency is highly suspected or demonstrated.

The patient with SLE must also receive a thorough preoperative pulmonary evaluation, including chest x-ray, pulmonary function test (PFT), and arterial blood gas analysis. PFT results often demonstrate a restrictive pattern in patients with SLE. Therefore the anesthetist should increase the inspiratory: expiratory ratio to 1:2.5 or 1:3 to reduce the potential for air trapping. The patient with SLE who demonstrates interstitial disease will likely have decreased diffusing capacity. Loss of diffusing capacity may prolong inhalational agent concentration changes and may prolong both induction and emergence as well. If the patient with SLE also has bronchiolitis, the PFT results may show an obstructive pattern. Postoperative ventilatory support may be necessary for the patient with significant pulmonary dysfunction. The anesthetist must communicate this possibility to the patient preoperatively.

S

Tyrosinemia

Definition

Tyrosinemia is an aminoacidopathy of tyrosine metabolism
with elevated serum and urinary tyrosine excretion and related
metabolites. Type I results in inhibition of some renal tubular
function. The renal implications are similar to the renal dysfunction
observed with Fanconi syndrome (see p. 132). Tyrosinemia is also
known as hereditary tyrosinemia type I (HTI).

Incidence

The overall incidence of tyrosinemia is estimated at 1:100,000.
Northern European populations demonstrate an approximate incidence of 1:8000, whereas the population of Quebec, Canada, demonstrates an incidence of 1:1846. There is no gender preference.

Etiology

HTI results from the homozygous, autosomal recessive inheritance of a genetic mutation on chromosome 15, loci q23-q25.
To date 30 distinct mutations at these loci have been documented.

Signs and Symptoms

- Anorexia
- Bloody stool
- Cabbage-like body odor
- Cirrhosis
- Diarrhea
- Diminished nutritional
  intake
- Epistaxis
- Failure to thrive
- Hepatic nodules
- Hepatomegaly
- Jaundice
- Lethargy
- Marked edema
- Melena
- Polyneuropathy
- Purpuric lesions
- Vomiting

Medical Management

Treatment of HTI is directed toward the patient's acute
hepatic decompensation, which may result in greatly reduced
or even absent critical coagulation factors. Replacement or

replenishment of inadequate and/or absent coagulation factors is necessary to prevent inordinate blood volume losses from even seemingly benign injuries.

The patient with HTI has some dietary restrictions. Specifically, the patient must minimize intake of phenylalanine and tyrosine to allow for only the essential daily requirements.

The child with HTI is typically critically ill on presentation. Stabilization is essential. Currently, surgical interventions are limited. Development of severe cirrhosis, hepatocarcinoma, or other hepatic lesion(s) may necessitate liver transplantation, but this extreme measure is typically a treatment of last resort.

Complications

- Abdominal crisis
- Hepatic cirrhosis
- Hepatocellular carcinoma
- Hepatoma
- Peripheral neuropathy
- Renal Fanconi syndrome (see p. 132)
- Renal tubular acidosis type 2
- Rickets secondary to renal tubular acidosis
- Seizures

Anesthesia Implications

Dehydration is a real risk at any time for the patient with tyrosinemia. As a result, the patient's NPO duration should be kept to the safest tolerable minimum time.

The patient being treated with diuretic therapy should also have an electrolyte level determined immediately before surgery, with attention focused on the potassium concentration. Potassium supplementation may be necessary and may cause a nonemergent and/or elective operative procedure to be delayed until the potassium concentration has been corrected.

Arterial blood gas analysis may be needed in conjunction with analysis of electrolyte levels to determine the current state of acid-base equilibrium. The patient may attempt to compensate by inducing a respiratory alkalosis. Anesthetists must watch for this possibility to ensure that the balance is not altered significantly, which could exacerbate the metabolic acidosis that arises as a result of the patient's altered respiratory pattern during general anesthesia. Adequate ventilation during general anesthesia may necessitate supplemental administration of sodium bicarbonate and should be guided by serial arterial blood gas analyses during anesthesia.

Because of the potential need for obtaining multiple blood samples, insertion of an arterial pressure line may be appropriate—even considerate—for the patient.

Liver function testing is of particular concern for the patient with tyrosinemia, especially one with concurrent Wilson's disease (see p. 355) or Fanconi syndrome (see p. 132).

Patients may be developmentally delayed and have significant speech impairment as a result of associated galactosemia. Therefore, extra effort and patience may be required of the anesthetist to foster patient understanding and cooperation before administering the anesthetic.

Because the patient's NPO status may be altered and renal failure is possible, general anesthesia should be induced via rapid sequence induction.

Selection of a volatile agent for maintenance of general anesthesia should be guided by the patient's degree of renal involvement or dysfunction. Regional anesthesia may be appropriate, but fluid resuscitation must be tempered by the degree of renal dysfunction that may be present.

Metabolism of various anesthesia-related medications, from nondepolarizing muscle relaxants to midazolam to opioid analgesics, may be altered as a result of the degree of the patient's liver dysfunction.

V

von Willebrand Disease

Definition

von Willebrand disease (vWD) is a bleeding disorder resulting from an autosomally inherited defect that causes a deficiency, or absence, of von Willebrand factor. This disease is associated with impaired platelet adhesion and epistaxis, as well as increased blood loss from trauma, surgery, menorrhagia, or postpartum bleeding.

Incidence

The incidence of this clinically significant disease is estimated at approximately 125:1,000,000. The incidence of severe vWD is estimated at approximately 0.5:1,000,000 to 5:1,000,000. There are no observed racial or gender predilections.

Etiology

vWD is an inherited defect in the von Willebrand factor gene, which is located on the short arm of chromosome 12. It is divided into three major types: Type I: partial quantitative deficiency; Type II: qualitative deficiency; and Type III: total deficiency. The types are differentiated by molecular mechanisms resulting from differences in the von Willebrand factor gene mutation and its expression.

Signs and Symptoms

- Delayed postsurgical bleeding
- Easy bruising
- Epistaxis
- Excessive menstrual bleeding
- Hematoma from relatively innocuous contact/ "trauma"
- Oral cavity bleeding
- Prolonged bleeding from minor trauma
- Severe hemorrhage after major surgery

Types of von Willebrand Disease

Type/Subtype	Description
Type I	Partial quantitive deficiency
Type II	Qualitative deficiency
Subtype IIA	Loss of large and medium multimers
Subtype IIB	Loss of large multimers via different mechanism than Type IIA
Subtype IIM	Interference in ability to bind factor VIII qualitative variants is associated with decreased platelet-dependent function but does not result from the absence of high molecular weight multimers
Subtype IIN	Defect in plasma von Willebrand factor causing interference
Type III	Complete deficiency of von Willebrand factor

Medical Management

There are two treatment options for the patient with vWD: desmopressin and/or transfusion therapy. The effectiveness of desmopressin depends on the type of vWD. For the patient with Type I, desmopressin is most effective. Desmopressin may triple or quadruple the plasma concentration of von Willebrand factor. For the patient with Type II, response to desmopressin is variable, depending on the subtype. Subtype IIA may have a strong but transient response with return to baseline within 4 hours. The patient with Subtype IIB should not receive trial administrations of desmopressin because of a predisposition to thrombocytopenia and potential thrombotic complications. For the patient with Type III, desmopressin has no effect because the patient is virtually devoid of von Willebrand factor. Platelet transfusion may be useful for a patient with vWD who is refractory to other therapies.

Cryoprecipitate and/or fresh frozen plasma may be used because each contains functional von Willebrand factor. However, their use is discouraged because both can result in transmission of viral disease from the donor. Achieving satisfactory plasma levels of von Willebrand factor with fresh frozen plasma transfusion requires a large volume to be infused, which is an additional reason why use of fresh frozen plasma is discouraged.

V

Complications

- Postoperative hemorrhage
- Transmission of viral disease via transfusion of cryoprecipitate or fresh frozen plasma, such as HIV/AIDS and hepatitis

Anesthesia Implications

The factor VIII concentration and bleeding times should be determined the week preceding the proposed surgery. Immediately before surgery, 1 to 2 hours a prophylactic infusion of desmopressin, 0.3 mcg/kg, should be administered. If the factor VIII and bleeding time baseline measurements are abnormal, they should be repeated after the desmopressin has been given. Desmopressin infusions should be continued daily until the surgical wound is healed. Factor VIII and bleeding times should also continue to be assessed until the wound is healed.

Because of the great potential for bleeding, unnecessary needle sticks should be avoided if at all possible. Attempts at intravenous access, intra-arterial pressure monitoring, or arterial blood gas analysis must be undertaken with great caution. Unsuccessful attempts require the anesthetist to hold pressure at the puncture site for a long time to minimize the bleeding and hematoma formation. Also as a result of the greater potential for bleeding and hematoma formation, regional anesthesia is relatively contraindicated. However, with appropriate prophylactic treatment using desmopressin, regional anesthesia can be undertaken with caution.

Wegener's Granulomatosis

Definition

Wegener's granulomatosis (WG) is the systemic vasculitis of small and medium arteries, venules, and arterioles. Large arteries may also be affected.

Incidence

WG is rare; the exact frequency is not known. Recent estimates of incidence put the occurrence at 1:30,000 to 1:50,000 individuals. The age of onset peaks at 40 to 50 years, and it appears equally in males and females, with a strong predilection for Caucasians (>97% of cases).

Etiology

The exact cause of WG is still unknown. Antineutrophilic cytoplasmic antibody (ANCA) has been detected in most cases, and the concentration seems to correlate with the severity of the disease.

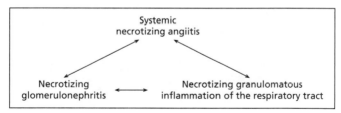

Triad of Physiologic Features of Wegener's Granulomatosis.

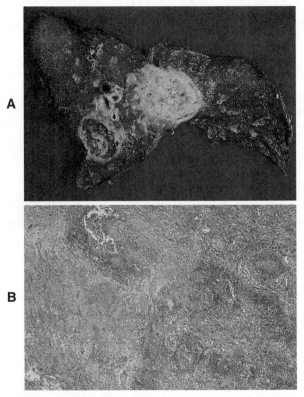

Wegener's Granulomatosis. The lung parenchyma contains two nodules showing central necrosis. *(From Damjanov I, Linder J: Pathology: A Color Atlas, St Louis, 2000, Mosby.)*

Signs and Symptoms

- Acute nephritis
- Acute renal failure
- Anorexia
- Arthralgia
- Atelectasis
- Conjunctivitis
- Corneal ulceration
- Cough
- Episcleritis
- Fatigue
- Fever
- Hemoptysis
- Malaise
- Night sweats
- Otitis media
- Pleural effusion
- Pleuritis
- Rapidly progressing glomerulonephritis
- Rhinorrhea
- Sinusitis
- Urine color change
- Weakness
- Weight loss

Medical Management

WG is treated with a combination of prednisone and cyclo-phosphamide. After control of WG is established, the predni-sone is tapered off over a 2-month period; cyclophosphamide is continued for another 6 to 12 months. The patient who does not tolerate the cyclophosphamide may respond more favorably to azathioprine, chlorambucil, or methotrexate. Methotrexate is not given to the patient with pulmonary hemorrhage or fulminate renal failure. Remission may be followed by reappearance of the disease. Relapses usually respond favorably to another regimen of prednisone and cyclophosphamide.

The patient with WG may suffer damage to the nose, subglottic region, trachea, and bronchial tree that may require surgical correction. The patient who progresses to renal failure should be qualified and considered for renal transplant.

Complications

- Acute renal failure
- Acute respiratory failure
- Blindness
- Chronic renal failure
- Deafness
- Massive hemoptysis
- Nasal septum perforation
- Neuropathy
- Saddle nose
- Tracheal stenosis

Anesthesia Implications

Pulmonary and renal effects of this disease must be assessed
before any proposed surgical intervention. Blood urea nitrogen
(BUN) and creatinine are hallmark preliminary indicators of
renal dysfunction.

Tracheal stenosis may be detected using pulmonary flow-
volume loop, which detects changes in tracheal caliber. Pulmonary function tests plus spirometry will help indicate whether
WG has produced a restrictive pulmonary disorder
or an obstructive pulmonary disease.

The patient with WG may have an unexpectedly difficult
airway. By outward appearance and cursory physical examination,
the patient may appear to have normal airway anatomy. However,
there may be a great amount of granulation tissue within the
nasal cavity. This highly vascular tissue may impede the insertion of either a nasal airway or passage of a nasotracheal tube.
Even if either of these airway devices is able to be inserted, the
granulation tissue may be significantly traumatized, resulting
in considerable blood loss. Unless absolutely required by the
proposed surgical procedure, use of nasal airway devices should
be avoided. The epiglottis and oropharynx may be covered
with a significant amount of granulation tissue or lesions that
may significantly impede placement of an oral endotracheal
tube. Even when the glottis is easily visualized, passage of
the tube may not be possible because of unforeseen tracheal
stenosis. When preparing to anesthetize a patient with WG,
the anesthetist should have a variety of sizes of endotracheal
tubes within immediate reach along with a difficult airway cart
containing numerous airway devices, particularly the laryngeal
mask airway (LMA), intubating LMA, and fiberoptic bronchoscope. Use of any of these devices to secure the patient's airway
may traumatize the granulation tissue and produce significant
bleeding, further obscuring an already cloudy scene. Finally, all
these possibilities may conspire to render the airway unsecur-
able, at which time emergent surgical intervention may be
required to establish the patient's airway.

The patient with WG is typically treated with relatively
long-term administration of corticosteroids. As a result, this
patient is likely to require perioperative coverage with corticosteroids.

Because WG can produce significant pulmonary sequelae, either as a restrictive or an obstructive disease, the patient is more prone to air trapping and barotrauma. During positive pressure ventilation, particularly mechanical ventilation, the inspiratory:expiratory ratio (I:E) should be prolonged to levels such as 1:2.5 or 1:3 to allow for better excursion, reduce or prevent air trapping and, thus, reduce or prevent barotrauma.

Regional anesthesia is a possibility for the patient with WG. However, before finalizing such a decision, a neurologic examination should be completed.

The medication and dosage of the neuromuscular blocking agent selected must be adjusted to account for the degree of renal dysfunction present as a result of the WG. Also, the degree of skeletal muscle wasting resulting from associated neuritis calls into question the use of succinylcholine; the prudent course would be to avoid administering succinylcholine.

If there is significant WG-related myocardial muscle and/or cardiac valve involvement, a "normal" concentration of the volatile anesthetics can give rise to an inordinate degree of myocardial depression. The concentration may thus need to be reduced. Other agents known to produce significant myocardial depression, such as propofol, are best avoided in favor of potentially less depressing drugs, such as ketamine or etomidate. The ECG should be closely observed for signs of significant myocardial depression. Direct monitoring of arterial blood pressure may be difficult, depending on the extent of arteritis present.

Chronic Symptoms of Wegener's Granulomatosis after Remission

- Chronic renal disease
- Cosmetic nasal deformity
- Hearing loss
- Hoarseness
- Tracheal stenosis
- Visual loss

The patient with WG may be leukopenic and anemic
as a result of taking the immunosuppressant cyclophosphamide.
Cyclophosamide also tends to reduce the available concentration of plasma cholinesterases, which may result in prolonged
response to succinylcholine and/or other plasma
cholinesterase–dependent drugs.

Williams Syndrome

Definition

Williams syndrome is a rare genetic disorder that results in hypercalcemia, cardiovascular anomalies, neurodevelopmental and/or behavioral problems, and development of distinct facial features.

Incidence

The incidence of Williams syndrome is estimated to be 1:20,000, without racial, ethnic, or gender predilection.

Etiology

Unequal meiotic crossover produces interstitial deletions—notably, a deletion on band 7q11.23 near the elastin gene has been found in almost every patient with Williams syndrome.

Signs and Symptoms

- Bladder diverticula
- Bowel diverticula
- Calcified valvular aortic stenosis
- Cataract
- Coronary insufficiency
- Delayed motor development
- Dental malocclusion
- Failure to thrive
- Flat malar area
- Flat nasal bridge
- Full lips
- Gait ataxia
- Hearing loss
- Hyperactivity
- Hyperacusis
- Hypersensitivity to loud sounds or certain types of sounds
- Hypertension
- Hypoplastic nails
- Kyphoscoliosis
- Long philtrum
- Lordosis
- Mental retardation
- Microcephaly
- Periorbital fullness
- Precocious puberty
- Progressive joint contractures
- Raspy/harsh voice
- Reduced binocular vision
- Retinal vascular tortuosity
- Severe dental disease
- Severe pulmonary stenosis
- Short stature
- Short, upturned nose

- Stellate irides (starburst appearance of iris)
- Strabismus
- Supravalvular aortic stenosis (SVAS)
- Urinary frequency
- Valgus deviation of hallices
- Ventricular hypertrophy with biventricular outflow tract obstruction
- Wide mouth
- Widely spaced teeth

Medical Management

Treatment of the patient with Williams syndrome is specifically designed in response to the clinical presentation. The syndrome is evident very early after birth. Typically initial interventions address the patient's failure to thrive, hypercalcemia, or a cardiac lesion. Nutritional manipulation may simultaneously treat failure to thrive and hypercalcemia by reducing vitamin D and calcium intake to achieve normal serum calcium levels and promote optimal growth patterns.

The patient with Williams syndrome should be monitored for development of hypertension. If hypertension does develop, it should be treated without delay.

Cardiac lesions are common in the patient with Williams syndrome. The most common such lesion is supravalvular aortic stenosis (SVAS), which is also the cause of the most frequent surgical intervention. The decision to initiate the surgical intervention depends on the patient's cardiac symptoms, the magnitude of the pressure gradient across the supraaortic obstruction, or the presence of ischemic changes on a stress test. SVAS tends to progress over time, requiring long-term cardiac assessments.

Complications

- Bladder diverticula
- Hearing loss
- Myocardial ischemia resulting from biventricular outflow tract obstruction
- Myocardial ischemia resulting from coronary insufficiency
- Ocular problems
- Progressive heart failure
- Progressive joint contractures
- Respiratory infection
- Severe dental disease
- Severe pulmonary stenosis
- Sigmoid diverticulitis
- Sudden death
- Supravalvular aortic stenosis

Anesthesia Implications

The patient with Williams syndrome may present a significant anesthesia challenge. Several organ systems are affected by Williams syndrome; most important to the anesthetist are the effects on the cardiovascular and renal systems as well as the effects produced on the patient's airway.

Williams syndrome patients are particularly prone to cardiac and cardiovascular anomalies, such as SVAS, peripheral branch pulmonary stenosis, and hypertension. The most disconcerting is SVAS (see Medical Management above). Before receiving any anesthetic, general or regional, the patient with Williams syndrome should undergo a very thorough cardiac evaluation. The anesthetist should obtain previous 12-lead electrocardiograms, echocardiograms, chest x-rays, and/or cardiac catheterization reports for comparison. Any of these reports not completed within the 12 months before the surgery date should be updated.

The anesthetist must strive to maintain the patient's normal or usual resting heart rate. Avoidance of bradycardia or tachycardia and significant reductions in the systemic vascular resistance (SVR) are most important, along with maintenance of normotension (as close to what is normal for the patient as possible). Because of the strong need to avoid these possible effects, general anesthesia is likely the most appropriate anesthetic choice. Regional anesthesia, specifically subarachnoid or epidural blockades, should be avoided because of the sympathectomy it produces, resulting in significant reductions in both SVR and systemic blood pressure. The cardiovascular system of the patient with Williams syndrome should be closely monitored. The anesthetist should consider using an arterial pressure catheter, central venous catheter, pulmonary artery catheter, and/or transesophageal echocardiography to be able to more fully evaluate the patient's cardiovascular stability perioperatively. The extent of the invasive monitoring will depend on the severity of the patient's cardiac dysfunction along with the nature of the proposed surgical intervention.

The patient with Williams syndrome is prone to micrognathia as well as loose and/or brittle teeth—a state of generalized poor dentition that is not reflective of his or her hygienic routine or dental care. The patient's airway should be assessed preoperatively. An underdeveloped mandible may indicate possible difficulty in securing the patient's airway.

Before obtaining consent for anesthesia, the anesthetist must fully advise the patient and/or parent or legal guardian (if the patient is a minor or mentally/intellectually incompetent) of the increased risk for dental trauma despite the anesthetist's care, skill, and/or experience during the necessary direct laryngoscopy. It is absolutely necessary that the anesthetist have the difficult airway cart immediately at hand before induction of anesthesia.

The patient with Williams syndrome frequently has some degree of intellectual deficit or mental retardation. The level of the patient's intellectual and emotional development must be strongly considered when deciding on premedication for anxiolysis. The anesthetist must also take into account the degree of cardiac dysfunction in the "equation" to determine the method, as well as magnitude, of premedication the patient should receive, if any. It may be most appropriate to have the parent or legal guardian accompany the patient until induction of general anesthesia is accomplished.

The patient's kidney function should be assessed preoperatively. Hypercalcemia and hypercalciuria may predispose the patient to renal calculus formation, along with urinary tract disorders. The patient's serum creatinine and blood urea nitrogen (BUN) levels should be obtained preoperatively for use as indicators of renal function.

The patient with Williams syndrome is predisposed to joint contractures, so the anesthetist must be acutely aware of these special needs when positioning the patient during surgery and anesthesia. Extra caution is necessary during the positioning process to ensure copious padding of extremities, bony prominences, and pressure points. Gelatin pads are preferable because they disperse pressure more effectively than do foam pads. The presence of any contractures may require considerable "creativity" on the anesthetist's part to fulfill these needs.

Wilson's Disease

Definition

Wilson's disease is an autosomal recessive, inherited, rare, progressive disorder in the metabolism of copper, characterized by excessive copper deposits in the brain, liver, and other tissues. These deposits result from excessive absorption of copper by the small intestines coupled with inadequate excretion of copper by the liver.

Incidence

The incidence of Wilson's disease varies according to the country and the rate of consanguinity. For example, the incidence in Japan is 1:30,000, whereas the incidence in Australia is 1:100,000.

Internationally there are estimated to be 10 to 30 million cases of Wilson's disease. The age of onset of liver manifestations peaks between 10 to 13 years, whereas neuropsychiatric illness onset ranges from 19 to 20 years. Females present fulminant cases more frequently than males by a 4:1 ratio.

Etiology

Wilson's disease is a result of an autosomal recessive inheritance of the Wilson's disease gene on chromosome 13; more than 40 mutations have been delineated.

Four Stages of Wilson's Disease	
Stage I	Initial copper accumulation by liver binding sites
Stage II	Acute copper redistribution within the liver and systemic circulation
Stage III	Chronic accumulation of copper in the brain, renal, and other nonhepatic tissues
Stage IV	Achievement of copper balance via chelation therapy

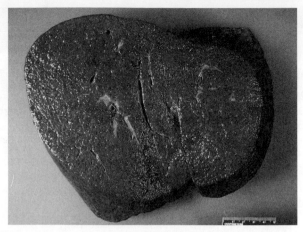

Wilson's Disease. Enlarged, firm, nodular appearing liver from a patient with *Wilson's disease who underwent liver transplant. (From Zitelli BJ, Davis HW: Atlas of Pediatric Physical Diagnosis, ed. 5, St. Louis, 2007, Mosby.)*

Signs and Symptoms

- Asymmetric tremor
- Ataxia
- Coombs-negative acute intravascular hemolysis
- Defective renal acidification
- Degenerative arthropathy
- Difficulty speaking
- Disinhibition
- Dystonia (rare)
- Excessive renal excretion of amino acids, glucose, fructose, galactose, pentose, uric acid, phosphate, and calcium
- Excessive salivation
- Flexion contractures (rare)
- Grand mal seizures (rare)
- Hemolytic anemia (rare)
- Impulsiveness
- Kayser-Fleischer rings
- Mask-like facies
- Osteopenia
- Personality changes
- Rigidity (rare)
- Self-injurious behaviors/ actions
- Spasticity (rare)
- Urolithiasis

Medical Management

Chelation therapy is the pharmacologic treatment of choice in Wilson's disease. The primary chelating agents are penicillamine and trientine.

Surgical interventions are limited. Portal hypertension may require transjugular intrahepatic portosystemic shunting (TIPS) or surgical decompression, particularly for the patient who has uncontrollable and/or recurrent variceal bleeding.

The only potentially curative intervention for Wilson's disease remains orthostatic liver transplantation. This most extreme measure is typically reserved for the patient in whom the effects of Wilson's disease progress to fulminant liver failure or the patient who develops end-stage liver cirrhosis.

Complications

- Coagulation abnormalities
- Fulminant liver failure
- Hepatic encephalopathy
- Hepatorenal syndrome
- Variceal bleeding

Anesthesia Implications

The first focus regarding the patient with Wilson's disease revolves around the function or dysfunction of the liver. Depending on the degree of liver dysfunction the patient has, virtually all the anesthesia-related medications may be anticipated to have a prolonged duration of effect. Cirrhosis and any attendant ascites may block either the production or retention of serum proteins and thus increase the bioavailability of many anesthesia-related medications, such as benzodiazepines or thiopental. Increased bioavailability can intensify drug effects. Therefore many of these anesthesia-related drugs should be given in reduced dosages.

Liver dysfunction secondary to Wilson's disease may hamper production of several clotting factors within the coagulation cascade or disable adequate utilization of vitamin K. Coagulation studies should be obtained preoperatively to determine whether the patient may benefit from administration of perioperative vitamin K and/or fresh frozen plasma to reduce inordinate blood volume losses. In addition, the patient with Wilson's disease should have a complete blood count (CBC) done preoperatively. The focus of the CBC should be on the platelet count because of the thrombocytopenia that penicillamine may induce. The patient may also require transfusion of platelets perioperatively—again, to reduce the amount of blood volume losses.

The abnormal metabolism of copper can produce copper deposition within brain tissue, resulting in various neuropsychiatric manifestations including ataxia, tremors, and dystonia. Because of these physical manifestations, obtaining intravenous access may be difficult and may require two people to establish, or may even necessitate placement of a central access intravenous line to ensure stability. The patient may be difficult, unable to fully cooperate as the result of confusion or other psychiatric manifestations secondary to the abnormal copper deposition in the brain tissue. The patient with Wilson's disease should not receive medications that exacerbate the extrapyramidal symptoms, such as metoclopramide, droperidol, promethazine, or prochlorperazine.

Renal function should be assessed before anesthesia. Urine output, along with blood urea nitrogen (BUN) and serum creatinine values, should be obtained to indicate the degree of renal dysfunction secondary to Wilson's disease. Because of the neuropsychiatric manifestations of this disease, the patient may be chronically dehydrated, resulting in a low urinary output as well as elevated BUN and serum creatinine concentrations. Altered renal function can significantly alter elimination of metabolic byproducts, active and inactive, of many anesthesia-related medications.

Wolff-Parkinson-White Syndrome

W

Definition

Wolff-Parkinson-White syndrome (WPW) is a paroxysmal tachycardia or atrial fibrillation associated with a preexcitation syndrome, characterized by a short P-R interval and a wide QRS complex with an early QRS vector or delta wave.

Incidence

WPW sydrome is estimated to affect approximately 0.15% to 0.2% of the general population. Males are more frequently affected than females.

Etiology

WPW syndrome results from accessory electrical connections between the atria and ventricles produced by anomalous embryonic myocardial tissue development bridging the septa. The connections produced allow electrical conduction via sites other than the atrioventricular node (AV node). Bypass tracts may be numerous, including atriofascicular, fasciculo-ventricular, intranodal, and nodoventricular. The most common bypass is an accessory AV pathway called a Kent bundle. Kent bundle conduction can occur anterograde and/or retrograde.

Signs and Symptoms

- Atrial fibrillation
- Auscultated crackles over lung fields
- Circus movement tachycardias (regular, generally narrow-complex tachycardias)
- Diaphoresis
- Dizziness
- Hypotension
- Palpitations
- Short P-R interval plus wide QRS complex with delta wave
- Weakness

Medical Management

Treatment regimens/interventions are dictated by the specific dysrhythmia(s). Immediate treatment measures should include obtaining intravenous access, electrocardiographic monitoring, blood pressure, and pulse oximetry. Supplemental oxygen is appropriate and especially important if the patient is hypoxic.

The primary goal in treatment of WPW atrial fibrillation is to induce prolongation of the anterograde refractory period. However, so-called conventional pharmacologic atrial fibrillation treatment—calcium channel blockers, β blockers, and digoxin—may be very deleterious and can cause rhythm deterioration that leads to ventricular fibrillation. The patient with WPW atrial fibrillation should receive synchronized cardioversion as the first-line intervention, particularly if the patient's condition is unstable. A hemodynamically stable patient may be treated medically, usually with a procainamide infusion.

Circus movement tachycardia should be treated so that the circus movement is broken and converted to a sinus rhythm. Cardioversion and adenosine are the common approaches used to achieve this goal. Adenosine is the first-line intervention when the patient is hemodynamically stable, but immediate cardioversion and full cardiac resuscitation equipment must be immediately on hand.

Complications

Any complications are attributable to the underlying condition.

Anesthesia Implications

The patient with WPW often presents for accessory pathway ablation. As such, pharmacologic interventions are frequently stopped to aid in inducing tachydysrhythmia. The patient is pharmacologically unprotected. Anxiolysis is important because it limits the chance of inducing a tachydysrhythmia in relatively uncontrolled surroundings, such as the patient's room, the elevator, and/or anesthesia holding room. Relatively heavy premedication is most helpful in achieving the desired degree of anxiolysis. An untoward initiation of atachydysrhythmia may be controlled using very short-acting agents, such as amiodarone, flecainide, propafenone, or sotalol, even though these drugs may interfere with the proposed ablation procedure.

General anesthesia, if necessary, may be best induced with a version of total intravenous anesthetic (TIVA) that is predominately opioid/benzodiazepine based or opioid/propofol based and has demonstrated a lack of interference with electrophysiologic parameters in the associated accessory conduction pathways. For ablation procedures, volatile anesthetic agents are relatively contraindicated because of their ability to increase refractoriness within the accessory and atrioventricular pathways. However, when a patient with WPW presents for a procedure other than ablation, it may be beneficial to use general anesthesia with volatile anesthetic agents to take advantage of the increase in the refractoriness to prevent incitement of perioperative tachydysrhythmias.

> ## Zenker's Diverticulum

Definition

Zenker's diverticulum is a rare pulsion disorder consisting of an esophageal mucosal herniation posteriorly between the cricopharyngeal muscle and the inferior pharyngeal constrictor muscle (at the junction of the pharynx and esophagus). It is actually a false diverticulum. Zenker's diverticulum is also called pharyngoesophageal diverticulum.

Incidence

The frequency of occurrence of Zenker's diverticulum in the United States and Europe is estimated to range from 0.01% to 0.11% of the population. The disorder is rare in the Middle East and Asia. Women are affected more frequently than men. The disorder is more often seen in the elderly, with age of onset typically occurring between 60 to 80 years.

Etiology

Zenker's diverticulum does not occur in any animal other than humans, so the etiology is poorly understood. Theoretically, the patient with Zenker's diverticulum has relaxation of the cricopharyngeal muscle that is poorly or improperly synchronized with the act of swallowing. The resultant increased pressure is cumulative, over time producing the posterior herniation of the esophageal mucosa between the inferior pharyngeal constrictor muscle and the cricopharyngeal muscle.

Signs and Symptoms

- Achalasia
- Aspiration pneumonia
- Esophageal spasm
- Esophagogastroduodenal ulceration
- Halitosis
- Hiatal hernia
- Mild-to-moderate weight loss
- Noisy deglutition
- Undigested food regurgitation
- Upper esophageal dysphagia
- Vocal changes

Medical Management

Management of Zenker's diverticulum consists entirely of surgical intervention. There are no absolute contraindications to surgical repair of Zenker's diverticulum. However, relative contraindications include (1) small diverticulum (<1 cm in diameter), which may be asymptomatic and may be followed by the surgeon pending development of symptoms and (2) the patient's ability to withstand the surgical procedure. The patient with strongly symptomatic disease is rarely denied surgical correction because there are many surgical approaches currently possible as well as the adaptability of anesthesia care for the chosen surgical approach.

Complications

- Aspiration
- Pneumonia
- Squamous cell carcinoma

Anesthesia Implications

Because of the nature of Zenker's diverticulum, surgery is the only definitive management. The anesthetist may need to exercise great flexibility and creativity in providing anesthesia. The anesthetist may be required to "share" the space with the surgical team. For example, when the surgical approach entails a rigid laryngoscopy by an otolaryngologist, the diverticulum may be stapled then excised. To facilitate such an approach, the anesthetist may need to place a smaller-than-usual endotracheal tube. Good muscle relaxation is an essential component of this surgical approach. The anesthetist may thus find it helpful to use an infusion of mivacurium because it can be rapidly discontinued, pharmacologically reversed, and has much less potential for residual effects. The anesthetist must consider the age of the patient with Zenker's diverticulum (the patient is usually quite elderly) and tailor the anesthetic plan accordingly.

Another surgical approach uses a relatively small incision in one side of the neck, dissects the structures and separates the esophagus from the surrounding musculature, then proceeds to the actual diverticulectomy. The considerations delineated above apply equally to this surgical approach, except the usual size endotracheal tube may be used without interference with the surgery.

Because of the nature of Zenker's diverticulum, the patient may be required to cease oral intake of liquids and solids for a longer time than usual for general anesthesia. This increased period without oral intake allows more time for the diverticulum to empty before surgery and anesthesia, thus reducing the potential for regurgitation and/or aspiration.

General anesthesia should be induced employing rapid sequence precautions despite the prolonged NPO status. However, the rapid sequence precautions should be modified to *exclude* cricoid pressure. Frequently, Zenker's diverticulum is located above the cricoid cartilage. As a result, application of cricoid pressure during the induction may expel any diverticulum contents. It may be more prudent to attempt to empty the diverticulum preoperatively, particularly if the pouch is large, regardless of the length of time the patient has been NPO. H_2 blockers, 5HT-3 antagonists, and/or antacids generally do not affect Zenker's diverticulum because its location is so distant from the stomach. Placement of a nasogastric or orogastric tube should be withheld because of the risk to the esophagus. Anesthesia should be maintained using short-acting agents to allow for a more rapid emergence at the conclusion of the procedure so that the patient quickly regains control of his or her airway reflexes. The anesthetist must also expect some delay in both induction and emergence as a result of the advanced age typical of patients with Zenker's diverticulum. Once sugery is completed and the patient has emerged from anesthesia, the oropharynx should be thoroughly suctioned to prevent aspiration of any expelled diverticulum contents at the time of extubation. Transfer to the post-anesthesia care unit should be accomplished with the head of the bed or stretcher elevated at least 30 degrees to reduce the potential for aspiration. In the post-anesthesia care unit, sedation should be kept to a minimum, also to reduce the possibility of aspiration. For more information on anesthesia implications, see Achalasia (p. 1).

Zollinger-Ellison Syndrome

Definition

Zollinger-Ellison syndrome (ZES) is a typical, intractable, possibly fulminating, peptic ulcer associated with extreme gastric hyperacidity.

Incidence

In the United States ZES is estimated to occur in 0.1% to 1% of all patients who have duodenal ulcers. Internationally the incidence of ZES varies; for example, Sweden reports 1:1,000,000 to 3:1,000,000; Ireland reports 0.5:1,000,000; and Denmark reports 0.1:1,000,000 to 0.2:1,000,000. ZES has been reported in all races. Males are slightly more likely to be affected than females by a ratio of 1.3:1. The mean age of onset is 43 years.

Etiology

The majority, about 75%, of ZES cases are the result of a non–β-islet cell, gastrin-secreting pancreatic tumor that stimulates the stomach's acid-secreting cells to their maximum output. The result is profound hyperacidity that can erode gastrointestinal mucosa to the point of ulceration. The remaining ZES cases result from an autosomal dominant familial syndrome, multiple endocrine neoplasia type I (MENI). In MENI, the primary tumor may be found in the duodenum, pancreas, or abdominal lymph nodes but may also be found in so-called ectopic areas, including the heart, ovaries, gallbladder, liver, or kidneys.

Signs and Symptoms

ZES

- Abdominal pain
- Diarrhea
- Gastrointestinal bleeding
- Heartburn
- Hypergastrinemia
- Hyperparathyroidism
- Malabsorption
- Nausea
- Pancreatic endocrine tumor
- Pituitary tumor(s)
- Vomiting
- Weight loss

MENI ZES
- Gastrinoma
- Hypercalcemia
- Hyperparathyroidism
- Nephrolithiasis

Medical Management

The treatment goals for ZES are (1) control hypersecretion of gastric acid, and (2) surgical resection of the causative tumor. The most effective pharmacologic intervention is the use of intravenous proton pump inhibitors. Proton pump inhibiting agents have demonstrated superiority to histamine (H_2)-blocking agents in achieving rapid control of gastric acid hypersecretion.

The causative tumor, usually a non–β-islet cell tumor of the pancreas, should be identified. Computed tomography (CT), somatostatin receptor scintigraphy (SRS), and endoscopic ultrasound are the most sensitive methods of identifying and localizing the tumor, as well as evaluating for evidence of metastasis of the tumor. Most patients with ZES (those with sporadic ZES) who do not demonstrate hepatic metastasis, should have the tumor surgically resected to reduce the possibility of liver metastasis. Surgical resection is more likely curative of a sporadic ZES tumor than it is for MENI/ZES, which is rarely cured by surgical intervention.

Complications

- Bowel obstruction
- Duodenal perforation
- Esophageal stricture
- Gastric carcinoids
- Hyperkalemia
- Hypovolemia
- Jejunum perforation
- Metabolic alkalosis

Anesthesia Implications

Before anesthesia, the patient with either form of ZES should be assessed for his or her state of hydration, electrolyte levels, and metabolic balance. ZES may be accompanied by profuse watery diarrhea, which can quickly produce significant dehydration, electrolyte imbalances (particularly hypokalemia), and metabolic alkalosis. From this preoperative evaluation, it may be necessary to initiate rather intense fluid resuscitation, with electrolyte supplementation, before inducing anesthesia. Induction of anesthesia with a patient significantly dehydrated can produce profound hypotension. A preoperative 12-lead electrocardiogram should be obtained to detect any dysrhythmic activity that might be related to or result from the diarrhea-induced electrolyte imbalance.

The patient with hepatomegaly and/or suspected liver metastasis should be screened preoperatively for coagulation ability as well as liver function. Liver metastasis can result in alterations in fat absorption, which can alter production of clotting factors and impair overall liver function. If these test results show significant alteration, the anesthetist should anticipate greater-than-normal blood volume losses, along with prolongation of action of many anesthesia-related medications.

The patient with ZES is medically managed with various combinations of H_2-receptor antagonists and proton pump inhibiting agents. The anesthetist must ensure continuation of those medications perioperatively. Intravenous ranitidine has demonstrated particular effectiveness in preventing intraoperative hypersecretion of gastric acid. The anesthetist should also place a nasogastric tube to evacuate the stomach and keep it as empty as possible throughout the surgery and anesthesia.

Finally, but very importantly, gastrin typically increases lower esophageal sphincter tone. However, gastroesophageal reflux disease (GERD) is commonly associated with ZES. The anesthetist should employ classic rapid sequence induction precautions to minimize the potential for reflux and aspiration. At the end of surgery, the patient should be almost fully awake with intact airway reflexes before the trachea is extubated. The patient should also be transported to the post-anesthesia care unit with the head of the bed or stretcher elevated a minimum of 30 degrees to reduce the potential for regurgitation and aspiration.

APPENDIX **A**

Antineoplastic Disease Chemotherapy Drugs

CLASSIFICATION: ALKYLATING AGENTS

Definition
Alkylating drugs become strong electrophiles by forming carbonium ion intermediates and other transitional complexes. The intermediate complexes form covalent links via alkylation of numerous cellular compound groups—for example: phosphate, amino, sulfhydryl, hydroxyl, carboxyl, and imidazole groups. The reactions result in alkylation of DNA, thereby producing chemotherapeutic and cytotoxic effects. By modifying the basic structure, alkylating agents alter reactivity, lipophilicity, biologic membrane active transport, and macromolecular attack sites, as well as DNA repair mechanisms. Each of these properties has a direct effect on the *in vivo* activity of a drug. DNA synthesis disruption/disturbance plus alteration of cell division are the most important pharmacologic actions of alkylating agents and are the basis for their therapeutic and toxic effects. Resistance to this class of drugs develops quickly via the following mechanisms:

1. Decrease in active transport
2. Increase in intracellular concentration(s) of neutrophilic compounds
3. Increase in DNA pathways of repair
4. Increase in metabolism of active drug forms

Untoward Effects
Bone marrow
- Acute immunosuppression
- Cellular and humoral immunity suppression

Leukemogenesis
- Neutropenia and/or anemia followed (about 4 years later) by acute nonlymphocytic leukemia

Mucosa
- Bacterial sepsis
- Intestinal denudation
- Ulceration of oral mucosa

Neurologic system
- Altered mental status
- Cerebellar ataxia
- Coma, seizures
- Nausea
- Vomiting

Other organs
- Alopecia
- Calcium and magnesium resorption difficulties
- Glycosuria
- Irreversible azoospermia
- Permanent amenorrhea
- Pulmonary fibrosis
- Renal failure
- Renal tubules acidosis
- Severe hemorrhagic cystitis
- Ulceration from extravasation
- Veno-occlusive disease of the liver

Type: Nitrogen Mustards
Drugs and dosages

Generic Name	Trade Name(s)	Typical Dosage Range
Chlorambucil	Leukeran	0.1-0.2 mg/kg/day initially 14 mg/m^2/day PO/IV for 5 days
Cyclophosphamide	Cytoxan	400 mg/m^2 IV for 5 days 500-1500 mg/m^2 every 21 or 28 days 100 mg/m^2 PO for 14 days
Ifosfamide	Ifex	50 mg/kg/day IV bolus dose 700-2000 mg/m^2/day for 5 days 2400 mg/m^2/day for 3 days 1200 mg/m^2/day continuous infusion for 5 days 5000 mg/m^2 single dose every 21 or 28 days
Mechlorethamine	Nitrogen mustard, Mustargen	0.4 mg/kg or 12-16 mg/m^2 IV as sole agent *Topical:* 10 mg in 60 mL of sterile water *Intracavitary:* 0.2-0.4 mg/kg

Continued

Type: Nitrogen Mustards—cont'd
Drugs and dosages—cont'd

Generic Name	Trade Name(s)	Typical Dosage Range
Melphalan	Alkeran, L-PAM, L-Phenylala-nine mustard, L-Serolysin	0.25 mg/kg/day PO for 4 days in combination with prednisone 2 mg/kg/day, repeat every 6 weeks 6 mg/m² PO for 5 days, repeat every 6 weeks 0.1 mg/kg PO for 2-3 weeks, then maintenance of 2-4 mg daily after bone marrow recovers

Commonly targeted diseases
- Acute and chronic lympho-cytic leukemia (see p. 13)
- Breast cancer
- Cervical cancer
- Hodgkin's disease
- Lung cancer
- Multiple myeloma
- Neuroblastoma
- Non-Hodgkin's lymphoma
- Ovarian cancer
- Primary macroglobulin-emia
- Soft tissue sarcoma
- Testicular cancer
- Wilms' tumor

Type: Ethylenediamines and Methylmelanines
Drugs and dosages

Generic Name	Trade Name(s)	Typical Dosage Range
Altretamine	Hexalen	4-12 mg/kg/day PO, in divided doses, for 21-90 days 240-320 mg/m² (6-8 mg/kg) PO daily for 21 days, repeat every 6 weeks
Thiotepa	Thioplex	8 mg/m² (0.2 mg/kg) IV daily for 5 days, repeat every 3-4 weeks 0.3-0.4 mg/kg IV every 3-4 weeks

Commonly targeted diseases
- Bladder cancer
- Breast cancer
- Ovarian cancer

Type: Methylhydrazine Derivative
Drugs and dosages

Generic Name	Trade Name(s)	Typical Dosage Range
Procarbazine HCl	Matulane	100 mg/m² PO daily for 7-14 days, repeat every 4 weeks

Commonly targeted diseases
• Hodgkin's disease

Type: Alkyl Sulfonate
Drugs and dosages

Generic Name	Trade Name(s)	Typical Dosage Range
Busulfan	Myleran	*Initial:* 4-8 mg/kg PO for 2-3 weeks *Maintenance:* 1-3 mg/m² PO daily or 0.05 mg/kg PO daily Titration depends on leukocyte count Drug is withheld when leukocyte count is <15,000/µL and may be resumed when leukocyte count reaches 50,000/µL

Commonly targeted diseases
• Chronic myelogenous leukemia

Type: Nitrosoureas
Drugs and dosages

Generic Name	Trade Name(s)	Typical Dosage Range
Carmustine	BCNU, BiCNU	75-100 mg/m² IV daily for 2 days 200-225 mg/m² every 6 weeks 40 mg/m²/day for 5 days, repeat every 6-8 weeks
Streptozocin	Zanosar	500 mg/m² IV daily for 5 days, repeat every 3-4 weeks 1500 mg/m² IV weekly

Commonly targeted diseases
• Hodgkin's disease
• Malignant carcinoid tumor
• Malignant pancreatic insulinoma
• Melanoma
• Non-Hodgkin's lymphoma
• Primary brain tumor

Type: Triazenes
Drugs and dosages

Generic Name	Trade Name(s)	Typical Dosage Range
Dacarbazine	DTIC-Dome	375 mg/m² IV every 3-4 weeks 150-250 mg/m²/day IV for 5 days, repeat every 3-4 weeks 800-900 mg/m² IV as a single dose every 3-4 weeks
Temozolomide	Temodar	*Patient who has received previous chemotherapy:* 150 mg/m²/day PO for 5 days, repeat every 28 days Adjust dosage to maintain absolute neutrophil count (ANC) of 1000-1500/mm³ with platelets at 50-100,000/mm³

Commonly targeted diseases
- Glioma
- Hodgkin's disease
- Malignant melanoma
- Melanoma
- Soft tissue sarcomas

Type: Platinum Coordination Complexes
Drugs and dosages

Generic Name	Trade Name(s)	Typical Dosage Range
Carboplatin	Paraplatin	*Singularly:* 360 mg/m² IV every 4 weeks *Combination:* 300 mg/m² IV with cyclophosphamide Delay for neutrophil count <2000/mm³ or platelet count <100,000/mm³ Adjust dosage downward for urine creatinine <60 mL/min
Cisplatin	Platinol-AQ	50-120 mg/m² IV every 3-4 weeks 15-20 mg/m² IV for 5 days, repeat every 3-4 weeks 15-50 mg/m² IV 1-3 times/week concurrent with radiotherapy to maximum cumulative dose of 50 mg/m²

Type: Platinum Coordination Complexes—cont'd
Drugs and dosages—cont'd

Generic Name	Trade Name(s)	Typical Dosage Range
Oxaliplatin	Eloxatin	*Day 1:* oxaliplatin 85 mg/m^2 IV in 200-250 mL D$_5$W plus leucovorin 200 mg IV in D$_5$W (each over 2 hours simultaneously in separate IV bags), followed by 5-FU 400 mg/m^2 over 2-4 minutes, then 5-FU 600 mg/m^2 in 200-250 mL D$_5$W over 22 hours *Day 2:* leucovorin 200 mg/m^2 IV over 2 hours, followed by 5-FU 400 mg/m^2 over 2-4 hours, then 5-FU 600mg/m^2 in 200-250 mL D$_5$W over 22 hours

Commonly targeted diseases
- Bladder cancer
- Colon cancer
- Esophageal cancer
- Lung cancer
- Ovarian cancer
- Testicular cancer

CLASSIFICATION: ANTIMETABOLITES

Definition
Antimetabolite drugs are structured in such a configuration that they appear to be essential metabolites necessary for the successful synthesis of DNA and RNA. The false metabolites are incorporated into the pathway(s) for DNA and RNA synthesis or act to block critical enzymes with the result being prevention of DNA synthesis and cellular death.

Untoward Effects
- Acute cerebellar syndrome
- Acute chest pain with ischemia
- Alopecia
- Anemia
- Anorexia
- Asthenia
- Ataxia
- Cirrhosis
- Defective oogenesis
- Defective spermatogenesis
- Dementia and coma (with intrathecal cytarabine administration)
- Dermatitis
- Erythematous/pruritic rash
- Fatigue
- Fetal toxicity
- Headaches

- Head-foot syndrome (erythema, desquamation, pain, and sensitivity to touch of palms and soles)
- Hepatic fibrosis
- Hyperthermia
- Increased pigmentation
- Interstitial pneumonitis
- Jaundice
- Leukopenia
- Mucosal ulcerations throughout the GI tract, may culminate in fulminant diarrhea, shock, and death
- Mucositis
- Myelopathy
- Myelosuppression
- Nail changes
- Nausea
- Nephrotoxicity
- Noncardiogenic pulmonary edema
- Optic neuritis
- Patchy inflammatory pulmonary infiltrates
- Pneumonitis
- Potential life-threatening infection
- Potential spontaneous hemorrhage
- Seizures
- Slowly progressive hemolytic uremic syndrome
- Slurred speech
- T-cell depletion
- Thrombocytopenia
- Tumor lysis syndrome

Type: Folic Acid Analogs
Drugs and dosages

Generic Name	Trade Name(s)	Typical Dosage Range
Methotrexate	Amethopterin, Mexate, Folex	*Low:* 10-50 mg/m^2 IV *Medium:* 100-500 mg/m^2 IV *High:* >500 mg/m^2 IV with leucovorin • 10-15 mg/m^2 intrathecal • 25 mg/m^2 IM
Pemetrexed	Alimta	500 mg/m^2 IV infused over 10 minutes every 21 days in conjunction with cisplatin 75 mg/m^2 IV over 2 hours Initiate cisplatin 30 minutes after pemetrexed

Commonly targeted diseases
- Acute lymphocytic leukemia (p. 13)
- Bladder cancer
- Breast cancer
- Choriocarcinoma
- Head cancer
- Lung cancer
- Mesothelioma
- Neck cancer
- Osteogenic sarcoma

Type: Pyrimidine Analogs
Drugs and dosages

Generic Name	Trade Name(s)	Typical Dose Range
5-Fluorouracil	Fluorouracil, Adrucil 5-FU, Efu-dex (topical)	12-15 mg/kg IV weekly 12 mg/kg IV for 5 days, repeat every 4 weeks 500 mg/m² IV weekly for 5 weeks *Hepatic infusion:* 22 mg/kg in 100 mL D_5W continuous infusion directly into hepatic artery over 8 hours for 5-21 days *Colon cancer:* variable *Head and neck cancer:* 1000 mg/m²/day continuous infusion for 4-5 days
Capecitabine	Xeloda	2500 mg/m²/day PO, divided into two doses per day with food for 2 weeks
Cytarabine Cytosine ara-binoside	Ara-C Cytosar-U	Disease dependent for dosage: *Leukemia:* 1000 mg/m²/day continuous infusion for 5-10 days 100 mg/m² IV or subcutaneous every 12 hours for 1-3 weeks *Head and neck cancer:* 1 mg/kg IV or subcutaneous every 12 hours for 5-7 days
Gemcitabine	Gemzar, Difluorode-oxycytidine	*Pancreatic cancer:* 1000 mg/m² IV over 30 minutes weekly up to 7 weeks then skip a week Treatment continues with weekly doses for 3 weeks and 1 week without *Non–small-cell lung cancer:* Given in conjunction with cisplatin • 4-week cycle: 1000 mg/m² IV over 30 minutes on days 1, 8, and 15, repeat every 28 days; the IV dose of cisplatin 100 mg/m² given on day 1 following gemcitabine • 3-week cycle: 1250 mg/m² IV over 30 minutes on days 1 and 8; cisplatin 100 mg/m² IV given day 1 after gemcitabine; repeat every 3 weeks

Commonly targeted diseases

- Acute lymphocytic leukemia
- Acute myelogenous leukemia
- Breast cancer
- Colon cancer
- Esophageal cancer
- Head and neck cancer
- Lung cancer
- Non-Hodgkin's lymphoma
- Ovarian cancer
- Pancreatic cancer
- Premalignant skin lesion
- Stomach cancer

Type: Purine Analogs
Drugs and dosages

Generic Name	Trade Name(s)	Typical Dosage Range
Cladribine	Leustatin, 2-CdA	0.09 mg/kg/day IV continuous infusion for 7 days
Fludarabine	Fludara	25 mg/m² IV infused over 30 minutes daily for 5 days, repeat every 28 days
Mercaptopurine	Purinethol, 6-MP	100 mg/m² PO daily for 5 days *Children:* • *Initial:* 70 mg/m² PO daily for induction • *Maintenance:* 40 mg/m² daily
Pentostatin	2'-Deoxycoformycin, NIPENT, Covidarabine	*Initial:* 500-1000 mL infusion of D₅ 0.45% saline, followed by additional infusion of 500 mL of fluid *Maintenance:* 4 mg/m² IV every other week

Commonly targeted diseases

- Acute lymphocytic leukemia (p. 13)
- Acute myelogenous leukemia (p. 14)
- Chronic lymphocytic leukemia
- Hairy-cell leukemia
- Small-cell non-Hodgkin's lymphoma

CLASSIFICATION: NATURAL PRODUCTS

Definition
Each type of drug in the class of natural products is derived
from compounds that occur in plants. The drugs interject
themselves into the mitotic cycle at various stages to arrest the
cycle, resulting in cell death.

Untoward Effects
Vinblastine (Velban, Velsar)
- Alopecia
- Aspermia
- Black, tarry stool
- Constipation
- Hypertension
- Increased urination
- Neurologic toxicity
- Sensitivity to sunlight
  (photophobia)
- Stomatitis

Vincristine (Oncovin, Vincasar)
- Agitation
- Alopecia
- Anorexia
- Arthralgia
- Confusion
- Constipation
- Depression
- Encephalopathy
- Fatigue
- Hallucinations
- Nausea
- Pain or difficult urination
- Paralysis
- Peripheral neuropathy
- Spinal nerve demyelin-
  ation (if intrathecal injec-
  tion occurs)

Vinorelbine tartrate (Navelbine)
- Alopecia
- Anemia
- Anorexia
- Chills
- Constipation
- Cough
- Fever
- Hives
- Irritation at the
  injection site
- Nausea/vomiting
- Pain
- Redness
- Sore throat
- Stomatitis
- Swelling
- Thrombocytopenia
- Tingling or numbness
  of the feet or hands

Type: Vinca Alkaloids
Drugs and dosages

Generic Name	Trade Name(s)	Typical Dosage Range
Vinblastine	Velban	0.1 mg/kg 6 mg/m^2 IV weekly
	Velsar	1.5-2.0 mg/m^2/day continuous infusion diluted in 1000 mL of D$_5$W or 0.9% saline for 5 days
Vincristine	Oncovin, Vincasar	0.4-1.4 mg/m^2 IV weekly, limited to 2 mg maximum per dose in the beginning
Vinorelbine tartrate	Navelbine	30 mg/m^2 IV weekly May be given in combination with cisplatin

Commonly targeted diseases
- Acute lymphocytic leukemia (p. 13)
- Breast cancer
- Hodgkin's disease
- Lung cancer
- Neuroblastoma
- Non-Hodgkin's lymphoma
- Rhabdomyosarcoma
- Testicular cancer
- Wilms' tumor

Type: Taxanes
Drugs and dosages

Generic Name	Trade Name(s)	Typical Dosage Range
Docetaxel	Taxotere	Dosages vary according to targeted disease Ranges from 60-100 mg/m^2 IV, usually every 3 weeks May be administered in conjunction with doxorubicin, cyclophosphamide, or cisplatin
Paclitaxel	Taxol, Onxol	*Untreated ovarian cancer:* • 135 mg/m^2 IV over 24 hours, then cisplatin 75 mg/m^2 every 3 weeks • Paclitaxel 175 mg/m^2 IV over 3 hours then cisplatin 75 mg/m^2 every 3 weeks *Treated ovarian cancer:* 135 or 175 mg/m^2 IV over 3 hours every 3 weeks *Node-positive breast cancer:* 175 mg/m^2 IV over 3 hours

Commonly targeted diseases
- Bladder cancer
- Breast cancer
- Head and neck cancer
- Lung cancer
- Ovarian cancer

Type: Epipodophyllotoxins
Drugs and dosages

Generic Name	Trade Name(s)	Typical Dosage Range
Etoposide	VP-16, VePesid, Etopophos	Dosages vary according to the targeted neoplasm Ranges from 50-200 mg IV daily for 3-5 days, repeat every 3-4 weeks *Bone marrow transplantation:* 750-2400 mg/m^2 IV (10-60 mg/kg) over 1-4 hours up to 24 hours in combination with other cytotoxic medications or total body irradiation
Teniposide	VM-26, Vumon	100 mg/m^2 IV weekly for 6-8 weeks 50 mg/m^2 IV twice a week for 4 weeks

Commonly targeted diseases
- Acute myelogenous leukemia (p. 14)
- Breast cancer
- Hodgkin's disease
- Non-Hodgkin's lymphoma
- Pediatric acute lympho-blastic leukemia
- Small-cell lung cancer
- Testicular cancer

Type: Camptothecins
Drugs and dosages

Generic Name	Trade Name(s)	Typical Dosage Range
Irinotecan	Camptosar, Camptothecin-II, CPT-11	125-150-350 mg/m^2 IV, depending on the neoplasm targeted May be given in conjunction with 5-FU and leucovorin

Continued

Type: Camptothecins—cont'd
Drugs and dosages—cont'd

Generic Name	Trade Name(s)	Typical Dosage Range
Topotecan	Hycamtin	1.25-1.5 mg/m^2 IV infused over 30 minutes for 5 days, repeat every 21 days

Commonly targeted diseases
- Colon cancer
- Lung cancer
- Ovarian cancer
- Small-cell cancer

Type: Antibiotics
Drugs and dosages

Generic Name	Trade Name(s)	Typical Dosage Range
Dactinomycin	Actinomycin D, Cosmegen	10-15 mcg/kg/day IV for 5 days every 3-4 weeks 15-30 mcg/kg/week 400-600 mg/m^2/day IV for 5 days
Daunorubicin	Cerubidine, Daunomycin HCl, Rubidomycin	30-60 mg/m^2/day IV for 3 days
Doxorubicin	Adriamycin	30-75 mg/m^2 IV every 3-4 weeks 20-45 mg/m^2 IV daily for 3 days *Bladder instillation:* 3-60 mg/m^2 *Intraperitoneal instillation:* 40 mg in 2 L of dialysate
Bleomycin	Blenoxane	5-20 units/m^2 IV/IM/subcutaneous weekly 10-20 units/m^2 IV/IM/subcutaneous twice per week
Epirubicin	Ellence, Farmorubicin(e), Farmorubicina, Pharmorubicin	60-100 mg/m^2 IV every 3-4 weeks Dosage depends on the targeted disease

Type: Antibiotics—cont'd
Drugs and dosages—cont'd

Generic Name	Trade Name(s)	Typical Dosage Range
Indarubicin	Idamycin, 4-Demethoxy-daunorubicin	12 mg/m^2 daily for 3 days combined with cytosine 100 mg/m^2 continuous infusion for 7 days 12 mg/m^2 daily for 3 days combined with cytosine 25 mg/m^2 IV push, followed by cytosine 200 mg/m^2 continuous infusion daily for 5 days
Mitomycin	Mitomycin C, Mutamycin, Mitozytrex	2 mg/m^2 IV daily for 5 days 5-20 mg/m^2 IV every 6 to 8 weeks *Bladder instillation:* 20-60 mg IV at a concentration of 1 mg/mL
Mitoxantrone	Novantrone	*Acute nonlymphocytic leukemia:* 12 mg/m^2 daily for 3 days, combined with cytosine arabinoside 100 mg/m^2/day continuous infusion for 7 days 10-14 mg/m^2 IV alone every 3-4 weeks
Plicamycin	Mithracin	*Testicular cancer:* 25-30 mcg/kg IV every other day until signs of toxicity occur *Hypercalcemia:* 25 mcg/kg IV single dose only

Commonly targeted diseases
- Acute leukemia (p. 13)
- Acute lymphocytic leukemia
- Acute myelogenous leukemia (p. 14)
- Breast cancer
- Choriocarcinoma
- Genitourinary cancer
- Hodgkin's disease
- Kaposi sarcoma
- Lung cancer
- Neuroblastoma
- Non-Hodgkin's lymphoma
- Osteogenic sarcoma
- Prostate cancer
- Rhabdomyosarcoma
- Soft tissue sarcoma
- Stomach cancer
- Testicular cancer
- Thyroid cancer
- Wilms' tumor

Illegal Drugs

DRUG NAME
Cocaine

Chemical Name
Benzoylmethylecgonine

Pharmacokinetic Data

Route of Intake	Onset of Action	Peak Effect
Inhaled	7 seconds	1-5 minutes
IV	15 seconds	3-5 minutes
Nasal	3 minutes	15 minutes
Oral	10 minutes	60 minutes

Half-Life
40-90 minutes, varies slightly with route of ingestion

Street Names (partial listing)
Angie, Aspirin, All-American drug, Babs, Beam, Bernie, Big C, Blow, C, California cornflakes, Candy sugar, Charlie, Coconut, Double bubble, Fast white lady, Friskie powder, Girlfriend, Happy dust, Happy trail, Henry VIII, Icing, Jelly, King, Lady snow, Late night, Love affair, Mosquitoes, Nose candy, Oyster stew, Pearl, Scorpions, Serpico 21, Sleigh ride, Star-Spangled powder, Teenager, Teeth, Twinkies, White horse, Wings, Witch, Yam, Yao, Yay, Zip

Signs of Acute Intoxication
- Dilated pupils
- Euphoria
- Increased blood pressure
- Increased heart rate
- Increased temperature
- Irritability
- Loss of appetite
- Mental clarity
- Peripheral vasoconstriction
- Reduced fatigue
- Restlessness

Associated Complications

- Agitation
- Airway burns
- Altered mental status
- Bronchiolitis obliterans organizing pneumonia
- Bronchospasm
- Cardiomyopathy
- Central retinal artery occlusion
- Chest pain
- Corneal ulcerations
- Decreased rapid eye movement (REM) sleep
- Depression
- Diarrhea
- Distorted perception
- Distractibility
- Dyspnea
- Dysrhythmias
- Epiglottitis
- Epistaxis
- Extrapyramidal phenomena
- Granulomatosis
- Hemoptysis
- Hemorrhagic stroke
- HIV/AIDS
- Hypertension
- Hyperthermia
- Intracranial hemorrhage
- Ischemic stroke
- Laryngospasm
- Myocardial ischemia or infarction
- Neurogenic pulmonary edema
- Neurogenic syncope
- Neuroleptic malignant syndrome
- New-onset seizures
- Optic neuropathy
- Paranoia
- Pneumomediastinum
- Pneumopericardium
- Pneumothorax
- Pulmonary edema
- Pulmonary hemorrhage or infarction
- Respiratory arrest
- Rhabdomyolysis
- Serotonin syndrome
- Sinusitis
- Tachypnea
- Torticollis
- Trismus
- Vomiting

B

DRUG NAME
Ecstasy

Chemical Name
3,4-methylenedioxymethamphetamine, MDMA

Pharmacokinetic Data

Onset of Action	Half-life	Peak Effect
30-60 minutes	12-34	90 minutes

Street Names (partial listing)
007s, 69s, Adam, Batmans, Bermuda triangles, Blue kisses, Blue lips, Candy Raver, Carebears, Dead road, Diamonds, Doctor, E, Egyptians, Elephants, Go, H-bomb, Herbal bliss, Igloo, Kleenex, Letter biscuits, Mercedes, Mitsubishi, Nineteen, Orange bandits, Pink panthers, Playboy bunnies, Red devils, Rolls Royce, Scooby snacks, Smurfs, Stars, Swans, Stacy, Tom and Jerries, Triple Rolexes, Wafers, Wheels, X, X-ing, XTC

Signs of Acute Intoxication
- Blurred vision
- Dry mouth
- Emotional warmth
- Enhanced sensations
- Euphoria
- Heightened feelings of empathy
- Little rushes of exhilaration
- Paresthesias
- Relaxation

Associated Complications
- Abdominal cramping
- Anorexia
- Anxiety
- Ataxia
- Autonomic instability
- Blurred vision
- Cerebral infarction
- Chest pain
- Diaphoresis
- Disseminated intravascular coagulation (DIC)
- Dysrhythmias
- Halos seen around objects
- Heart failure
- Hypertension
- Hypertensive crisis
- Hyperthermia
- Hyponatremia

- Nausea
- Palpitations
- Piloerection
- Renal failure
- Seizures
- Serotonin syndrome
- Stroke
- Subarachnoid hemorrhage
- Syncope
- Syndrome of inappropriate antidiuretic hormone (SIADH)
- Tachycardia
- Vomiting

B

DRUG NAME
Heroin

Chemical Name
Diacetylmorphine, diamorphine

Pharmacokinetic Data

Route of Ingestion	Onset of Action	Peak Effect
IV	1-2 minutes	10 minutes
IM, nasal	15-30 minutes	30 minutes

Half-Life
15-30 minutes

Street Names (partial listing)
Al Capone, Aunt Hazel, Ballot, Bart Simpson, Big H, Big Harry, Bin laden, Black eagle, Blows, Blue bag, Bozo, Brown sugar, Chip, Choco-fan, Cotic, Diesel, Dr. Feelgood, Eighth, Foil, Gallup, George, Goat, H, Hard candy, Hazel, Horse, Jerry Springer, Joy, Joy flakes, Little boy, Mexican horse, Muzzle, Nice and Easy, Number 4, Number 8, Nurse, Old navy, Old Steve, Peg, Poppy, Predator, Rambo, Reindeer dust, Salt, Spider, The Beast, Thunder, Train, White nurse, Witch-hazel, Z, Zoquete

Signs of Acute Intoxication
- Constipation
- Contentment
- Dreamlike state
- Dulled emotions
- Euphoria
- Itchiness
- Loss of appetite
- Nausea
- Pain relief
- Slow pulse
- Slow, shallow respirations
- Sweating
- Unconsciousness
- Vomiting
- Warmth
- Well-being

Associated Complications

- Aspiration pneumonitis
- Atelectasis
- Brain abscess
- Cellulitis
- Coma
- Endocarditis
- Extracerebral hematoma
- Fungal infections
- Granulomatosis
- Hepatitis
- HIV/AIDS
- Intracerebral hematoma
- Leukoencephalopathy
- Mycotic aneurysm
- Necrotizing fasciitis
- Noncardiogenic pulmonary edema
- Osteomyelitis
- Pneumomediastinum
- Pneumonia
- Pneumoperitoneum
- Pneumothorax
- Pulmonary hypertension
- Respiratory arrest
- Respiratory depression
- Rhabdomyolysis
- Seizures
- Sepsis
- Septic pulmonary emboli
- Stroke
- Suppurative thrombophlebitis
- Tuberculosis
- Valvular insufficiency

B

DRUG NAME
LSD

Chemical Name
Lysergic acid diethylamide

Pharmacokinetic Data

Route of Ingestion	Onset of Action	Peak Effect	Duration
Oral	30-90 minutes	3-5 hours	8-12 hours

Half-Life
175 minutes

Street Names (partial listing)
100s, 25s, Acid, Animal, Barrels, Birdheads, Black stars, Blue moons, Blue mists, California sunshine, Chocolate chips, Coffee, Doses, Dots, Elvis, Felix the Cat, Ghost, Hawaiian sunshine, Loony Toons, Lime acid, Mighty Quinn, Owsley, Pane, Potato, Rainbow, Snowmen, Strawberry fields, The Hawk, Ticket, Timothy Leary, Wedge, White Lightning, Yellow submarine, Zen

Signs of Acute Intoxication
- Diarrhea
- Distortion of time passage
- Feeling of "oneness with the universe"
- Feeling of inner tension
- Halos seen around objects
- Hyperactive reflexes
- Hypertension
- Illusions/hallucinations (visual, auditory, and sensory)
- Mild pyrexia
- Multiple, simultaneous emotions (depression, euphoria, joy, rage, terror, or panic)
- Piloerection
- Profound mydriasis
- Seizures
- Shapes blend/melt together
- Tachycardia
- Trail behind moving objects
- Tremors
- Vomiting

B

Associated Complications

- Coagulopathy
- Coma
- Exacerbation of preexisting psychiatric disorders
- Flashes of color
- Geometric hallucinations
- Hyperglycemia
- Hyperthermia
- Persistent/recurrent affective disorders
- Respiratory arrest
- Seizures

B

DRUG NAME
Marijuana

Chemical Name
Delta-l-tetrahydrocannabinol (THC) (the most powerful psychoactive substance)

1-*trans*-delta-9-tetrahydrocannabinol (substance believed responsible for mental effects)

More than 100 substances are released by burning

Pharmacokinetic Data

Route of Ingestion	Onset of Action	Peak Effect	Duration
Inhaled	A few minutes	1-2 hours	6-12 hours
Oral	30 minutes	1-2 hours	6-12 hours

Half-Life
4 hours

Street Names (partial listing)
Acapulco red, African, Airplane, Baby, Babysitter, Bar, Bash, Blonde, C. S., Canadian black, Cest, Charge, Chicago green, Dew, Ding, Ditch , Duby, Endo, Feeling, Firewood, Flower, Ganga, Gash, Giggle weed, Gold star, Hair cut, Hay, Herb, Indian boy, Jane, Jay, Jolly green, Kansas grass, KB, Key, L. L., Laughing grass, Lima, M. J., Macaroni, Meg, Mooster, Nigra, O. J., Pat, Pin, Queen Ann's lace, Railroad weed, Red bud, Red cross, Scrub, Scissors, Snap, Stack, Tex-Mex, Thumb, Viper's weed, Wake and Bake, Wheat, White Russian, Yellow submarine, Zambi

Signs of Acute Intoxication
- Drowsiness
- Dry mouth
- Euphoria
- Increased appetite
- Paradoxical hyperalertness
- Perception alterations
- Reddened eyes
- Relative uncoordination
- Relaxation
- Slowing of time perception
- Sluggishness
- Subjective feeling of well-being and/or grandiosity

Uncommon Effects

- Disorientation
- Dysphoria
- Hallucinations
- Illusions

- Memory impairment
- Mood lability
- Panicked feeling
- Paranoia

Associated Complications

- Abnormal spermatogenesis
- Cerebral atrophy
- Chronic obstructive pulmonary disease
- Complications associated with concurrent abuse of other substances
- Decreased sperm count

- Intoxicated infants (breastfed)
- Low-birth-weight infants
- Lung cancer
- Orthostatic hypotension
- Seizures
- Tachycardia

B

DRUG NAME

Mescaline; peyote (from the peyote cactus, *Lophophora williamsii*)

Chemical Name
3,4,5-trimethoxyphenethylamine

Pharmacokinetic Data

Route of Ingestion	Onset of Action	Duration of Effect
Oral	30 minutes-2 hours	8-12 hours

Half-Life
Approximately 90-120 minutes

Street Names (partial listing)
Buttons, Cactus, Cactus head, Mescal, Mese, Peyote, Topi

Signs of Acute Intoxication
- Ataxia
- Blurred vision
- Diaphoresis
- Dizziness
- Euphoria
- Hallucinations
- Nausea
- Numbness
- Pupil dilation
- Salivation
- Sensations of warm and cold
- Swatting
- Sweating
- Temporary splitting/ destruction of ego
- Trembling
- Uncontrollable laughter
- Vomiting

Associated Complications
- Hypertension
- Hyperthermia
- Psychosis
- Serotonin syndrome
- Tachycardia

DRUG NAME
Methamphetamine

Chemical Name
Methamphetamine hydrochloride

Pharmacokinetic Data

Route of Ingestion	Onset of Action	Peak Effect
IV or IM	2 minutes or less	≈30 minutes
Oral/vaginal	20-70 minutes	2-3 hours

Half-Life
10-20 hours, depending on urine pH

Street Names (partial listing)
Beannies, Black beauty, Blue devils, Chicken feed, Cinnamon, Clear, Desocsins, Desogtion, Fast, Geep, Getgo, Granulated Orange, Load of Laundry, Meth, Nazimeth, OZs, Pink, Redneck cocaine, Scootie, Sketch, Spackle, Tick tick, Wash, White cross, Work, Yellow bean, Yellow powder

Signs of Acute Intoxication
- Aggression
- Agitation
- Altered self-esteem
- Euphoria
- Excitation
- Increased alertness
- Increased sexual appetite
- Intensified emotions
- Psychotic behavior

Associated Complications
- Acute noncardiogenic pulmonary edema
- Acute toxic psychosis
- Agitation
- Anxiety
- Atrial dysrhythmias
- Cerebral edema
- Cerebral vasculitis
- Chest pain
- Clonus
- Coma
- Confusion
- Death
- Delusions
- Despondent affect
- Dyspnea
- Emotional lability
- Gastrointestinal ulcers
- Hallucinations
- Hepatitis B
- Hepatitis C
- HIV/AIDS

- Insomnia
- Ischemia
- Ischemic colitis
- Myocardial infarction
- Palpitations
- Paranoia
- Pneumomediastinum
- Pneumopericardium
- Pneumothorax
- Pulmonary hypertension
- Renal necrotizing angiitis
- Respiratory failure
- Rhabdomyolysis
- Seizures
- Spontaneous abortion
- Spontaneous cerebral hemorrhage
- Stroke
- Suicidal ideation
- Tachycardia
- Teratogenesis
- Ventricular dysrhythmias
- Wheezing

DRUG NAME
PCP (an arylcycloalkylamine)

Chemical Name
Phenylcyclohexylpiperidine; phencyclidine

Pharmacokinetic Data

Route of Ingestion	Onset of Action	Peak Effect	Duration of Action
Inhaled/IV	1-5 minutes	1-4 hours	4-6 hours
Oral/nasal (snorted)	30 minutes	1-4 hours	4-6 hours

Half-Life
7-46 hours; average of 21 hours

Street Names (partial listing)
Amoeba, Angel dust, Aurora borealis, Blue madman, Boat, Crazy Eddie, Detroit pink, Embalming fluid, Energizer, Flakes, Gorilla biscuits, Green tea, Hog, K, Kaps, KJ, Krystal joint, Lemon 714, Little ones, Magic, Mintweed, New magic, Peace pill, Peep, Pits, Rocket fuel, Sheets, Spores, STP, Tic Tac, Titch Wack, White Horizon, Yellow fever, Zombie Weed

Signs of Acute Intoxication
Vary according to blood levels

Blood Level	Symptoms
20-30 ng/mL	Hyperactivity, impaired attention, irritability, mood elevation, sedation
>30 ng/mL	Parestheslas, progressive ataxia, psychosis
100 ng/mL	Hyperreflexia, hypertension, hyperthermia, stimulant effects
>100 ng/mL	Death is possible, stupor, seizures

Associated Complications

- Acute hypertension
- Anxiety disorder
- Depression
- Flashbacks
- Kidney disease
- Prolonged psychosis
- Rhabdomyolysis
- Schizophrenia

Normal Pulmonary Function Tests and Arterial Blood Gas Values

Pulmonary Function Test	Accepted Normal Values
Vital capacity (VC)	60-70 mL/kg
Tidal volume (V_T)	6-8 mL/kg
Minute ventilation	80 mL/kg
Functional residual capacity (FRC)	28-32 mL/kg
Forced expiratory volume in 1 second (FEV_1)	>75%
Forced vital capacity (FVC)	60-70 mL/kg
Deadspace volume (V_{DS})	2 mL/kg
FEV_1/FVC	>75%
Residual volume	16 mL/kg
Closing capacity	23 mL/kg
Total lung capacity (TLC)	86 mL/kg

Arterial Blood Gas Values	Accepted Normal Values
pH	7.35-7.45
$Paco_2$	35-45 mm Hg
Pao_2	90-100 mm Hg
Sao_2(%)	95%-100%
Bicarbonate	22-26 mEq/L

Treatment of Anaphylaxis

Mild Reaction

- Discontinue the suspected causative agent
- Diphenhydramine 25-100 mg IV or IM

Moderate to Severe Reaction

- Discontinue the suspected causative agent
- Give 100% oxygen via mask with ventilatory support at hand
- Consider intubation
- Initiate fluid resuscitation: Lactated Ringer's solution 1-2 L initially
- Administer α-adrenergic agents for hypotension:
  - Epinephrine 5-10 mcg IV bolus or 0.05-0.1 mcg/kg/min continuous infusion
  - Norepinephrine 0.5-30 mcg/min infusion for systolic blood pressure <70 mm Hg
  - Dopamine 5-15 mcg/kg/min
  - Dobutamine 2-20 mcg/kg/min
- Bronchodilators to open constricted airway passages
  - Aminophylline 5-6 mg/kg
- Histamine-1, histamine-2 (H_1/H_2)-blockers: ranitidine 50-150 mg IV or cimetidine 300 mg IV
- Corticosteroids: hydrocortisone up to 200 mg IV or methylprednisolone 1-2 mg/kg IV

Anesthesia Drugs Metabolized by the Liver

- Alfentanil
- Atropine
- Bupivacaine
- Dexmedetomidine
- Ephedrine
- Etidocaine
- Etomidate
- Fentanyl
- Hydromorphone
- Ketamine
- Ketorolac
- Lidocaine
- Meperidine
- Mepivacaine
- Methohexital
- Midazolam
- Morphine
- Neostigmine
- Phenylephrine
- Prilocaine
- Propofol
- Rocuronium
- Ropivacaine
- Scopolamine
- Sufentanil
- Thiopental
- Vecuronium

Anesthesia Drugs Significantly Protein Bound

Drug	% Protein Bound
Propofol	95%–99%
Dexmedetomidine	94%
Morphine	35%
Meperidine	85%
Midazolam	97%

Rare Syndromes

Albright syndrome: Consists of polyostotic fibrous dysplasia, patchy dermal pigmentation, and endocrine dysfunction.

Antley-Bixler syndrome: A rare genetic disorder primarily characterized by distinctive craniofacial malformations along with skeletal abnormalities. The disorder is associated with craniosynostosis, prominent forehead, midfacial hypoplasia, proptosis, radiohumeral or radioulnar synostosis, arachnodactyly, bowing of the femur, and joint contractures.
Synonyms: Craniosynostosis; multisynostotic osteodysgenesis with long bone fractures; radial-humeral synostosis; trapezoidocephaly–multiple synostosis syndrome

Apert syndrome: A genetic defect classified as a craniofacial/limb abnormality. This disorder is characterized by craniosynostosis, retruded midface, fused fingers, and fused toes.
Synonyms: Acrocephalosyndactyly

Bickers-Adams syndrome: An X-linked form of hydrocephalus, responsible for 7% of cases of hydrocephalus in males, characterized primarily by stenosis of the aqueduct of Sylvius and severe mental retardation.

Bowen-Conradi syndrome: A rare, congenital genetic disorder characterized by intrauterine growth retardation, failure to thrive, craniofacial malformations, restricted joint movements, clinodactyly or camptodactyly of the fifth fingers, foot deformities, and/or cryptorchidism (in males). Some infants may have renal, brain, and/or other malformations.
Synonyms: Bowen-Hutterite syndrome; Bowen-Conradi-Hutterite syndrome; Hutterite syndrome, Bowen-Conradi type

Castleman's disease: A rare disorder characterized by systemic lymph node tissue benign tumors, most frequently found in the chest, stomach, and/or neck, but also may be found in the axilla, pelvis, and pancreas. There are three types: (1) hyaline-vascular, (2) plasma cell, and (3) generalized or multicentric. Hyaline-vascular type accounts for about 90% of all cases and is frequently asymptomatic. Plasma cell type may be associated with fever, weight-loss, skin rash, early red blood cell destruction, and/or hypergammaglobulinemia. Generalized or multicentric cases may exhibit hepatosplenomegaly.
Synonyms: Angiofollicular lymph node hyperplasia; angiomatous lymphoid; Castleman tumor; giant benign lymphoma; giant lymph node hyperplasia; hamartoma of the lymphatics

Cayler syndrome: An extremely rare congenital disorder characterized by congenital heart defects and underdevelopment or absence
of one of the muscles controlling lower lip movement—either
hypoplasia or agenesis of the depressor anguli oris muscle. Associated congenital heart defects include ventricular septal defect, atrial
septal defect, and/or tetralogy of Fallot. Microcephaly, micrognathia, microphthalmos, and/or mental retardation may occur in
some rare cases.

Synonyms: ACF with cardiac defects; asymmetric crying facies with
cardiac defects; Cayler cardiofacial syndrome; hypoplasia of the
depressor anguli oris muscle with cardiac defects

Chemke syndrome: A rare genetic, multisystem disorder characterized
by muscle disease and brain and eye abnormalities. Specific symptoms and their severity vary with each case. The most consistent
characteristics are lissencephaly, cerebellum and brainstem abnormalities, eye development abnormalities, and congenital muscular
dystrophy.

Synonyms: COD; COD-MD syndrome; cerebro-ocular dysgenesis;
cerebro-ocular dysplasia–muscular dystrophy syndrome; *h*ydroceph-
alus, *a*gyria, and *r*etinal *d*ysplasia (HARD) syndrome; HARD +/−
E syndrome; Pagon syndrome; WWS; Walker Warburg syndrome;
Warburg syndrome

Coats' disease: A rare disorder characterized by abnormal development of retinal blood vessels that may result in vision loss and retinal
detachment; usually affects only one eye, but rarely in both eyes.

Synonyms: Coats syndrome; retinal telangiectasis

Conotruncal anomaly face syndrome: A genetic disorder characterized by more than thirty features, including cleft palate, congenital
heart defects, facial abnormalities, learning difficulties, speech and
feeding problems. The disorder results from a deletion of a small
segment of chromosome 22.

Synonyms: Craniofacial syndrome; DiGeorge syndrome; Shprintzen
syndrome; velocardiofacial syndrome

Crouzon syndrome: A rare genetic disorder caused by mutations
of the FGFR2 or FGFR3 gene. The disorder is characterized by
flattened top and back of the head, flattened forehead and temples,
midfacial abnormalities, beaked-like nose, compression of nasal
passages, large protruding lower jaw, high-arched/narrow palate
or cleft palate, hearing loss, middle ear deformities, absence of ear
canals, Meniere's disease, vision problems, scoliosis, crossed eyes,
headaches, fused joints, and acanthosis nigricans.

Synonyms: Craniofacial dystosis; craniostenosis Crouzon type;
Crouzon craniofacial dystosis

Dandy-Walker malformation: A rare congenital malformation of the brain characterized by a cystic fourth ventricle that interferes with normal cerebrospinal fluid circulation through the foramina of Magendie and Luschka, motor delays, learning problems, and congenital hydrocephalus.

Synonyms: Dandy-Walker cyst; Dandy-Walker deformity; DWM; Dandy-Walker syndrome; Dandy-Walker type; internal Dandy-Walker type hydrocephalus; noncommunicating hydrocephalus; Luschka-Magendie foramina atresia

Faciocardiomelic syndrome: A very rare, congenital syndrome described only one time in which three siblings exhibited low birth weight, microretrognathia, microstomia, microglossia, hypoplasia of the radius and ulna with radial deviation of the hands, simian creases, hypoplasia of the first and fifth fingers, hypoplasia of the fibula and tibia with talipes and wide space between the first and second toes, and severe left heart malformations. This disorder is believed to be the cause of demise of the three reported siblings.

Synonyms: Faciocardiomelic dysplasia lethal

FG syndrome: An uncommon hereditary disorder that affects males and is characterized by mental retardation, imperforate anus, abnormal placement of the anus, constipation, hypotonia, a large head, and deafness (in some patients).

Synonyms: Opitz-Kaveggia syndrome

Grisel syndrome: A unilateral or bilateral subluxation of the C_1 on C_2 vertebrae associated with an infectious condition in the head or neck.

Heiner syndrome: A pulmonary disease produced by a food hypersensitivity, predominately to cow's milk; it is characterized by cough, wheezing, hemoptysis, nasal congestion, dyspnea, recurrent otitis media, recurrent fever, anorexia, vomiting, colic or diarrhea, hematochezia, failure to thrive, and pulmonary infiltrates.

Henoch-Schönlein purpura: A rare capillary inflammatory disease that is usually self-limiting, characterized by headache, fever, loss of appetite, abdominal cramping pain, joint pain, and petechial purpura.

Synonyms: Allergic purpura; allergic vasculitis; anaphylactoid purpura; HSP; hemorrhagic capillary toxicosis, Henoch's purpura; leukocytoclastic vasculitis; nonthrombocytopenic idiopathic purpura; peliosis rheumatica; rheumatic purpura; Schönlein's purpura; Schönlein-Henoch purpura

Marden-Walker syndrome: A rare, autosomal recessive inherited connective tissue disorder most frequently affecting males, characterized by a distinct facial expression, cleft or high-arched

palate, micrognathia, fixed bone joint position, growth delay, and
muscle spasticity.
Synonyms: Connective tissue disorder, Marden-Walker type;
MWS

Meckel syndrome: A rare, autosomal recessive inherited disorder characterized by multisystem abnormalities; three classic symptoms are:
1. Occipital encephalocele
2. Polycystic kidneys
3. Polydactyly
Children with this syndrome may have craniofacial abnormalities as
well as abnormalities of the liver, lungs, and genitourinary tract.
Synonyms: Dysencephalia splanchnocystica; Gruber syndrome;
MES; Meckel-Gruber syndrome; MKS

Mietens syndrome: A very rare, recessive genetic disorder characterized by multiple pterygia, cystic hygroma, hypoplastic heart and
lungs, skeletal abnormalities, facial anomalies, and growth retardation.

Opitz-G/BBB syndrome: A genetic disorder that may or may not be
apparent at birth. There are distinctive craniofacial malformations,
including ocular hypertelorism; cleft lip; cleft palate; palpebral
fissures; prominent epicanthal folds; or wide, flat nasal bridge.
Affected males may have cryptorchidism, bifid scrotum, and/or
hypospadias. Other possible symptoms include: tracheal
malformations, pharyngeal malformations, laryngeal malformations,
pulmonary hypoplasias, dysphagia, dyspnea, imperforate anus,
hypoplasia or agenesis of the corpus callosum, renal defects,
cardiac defects, or mental retardation.
Synonyms: BBBG syndrome; hypertelorism with esophageal
abnormalities and hypospadias; hypertelorism-hypospadias
syndrome; hypospadias-dysphagia syndrome; Opitz BBB syndrome;
Opitz BBB/G compound syndrome; Opitz BBBG syndrome;
Opitz-Frias syndrome; Opitz-G syndrome; Opitz hypertelorism-
hypospadias syndrome; Opitz oculogenitolaryngeal syndrome;
Opitz syndrome; telecanthus-hypospadias syndrome

Pfeiffer syndrome: A very rare genetic disorder characterized by
craniofacial abnormalities, distinctive malformations of the
fingers and toes, craniosynostosis, acrocephaly, syndactyly,
turribrachycephaly, midface hypoplasia, small nose with a flattened
bridge, ocular hypertelorism, hypoplastic maxilla, relative
mandibular prognathism, and/or dental abnormalities.
Synonyms: Acrocephalosyndactyly type I, subtype I; acrocephalosyndactyly V (ACSS or ACS V), subtype I; classic type Pfeiffer
syndrome; Noack syndrome, type I

Roberts syndrome: A rare genetic disorder characterized by pre- and postnatal growth deficiency, malformations of the arms and legs, craniofacial abnormalities, and mental retardation (in some cases). Limb abnormalities may range from tetraphocomelia to less severe degrees of limb reduction. Craniofacial abnormalities may include microbradycephaly, bilateral cleft lip, cleft palate, hypoplastic nasal alae, and/or dysplastic ears.

Synonyms: Hypomelia-hypertrichosis-facial hemangioma syndrome; pseudothalidomide syndrome; SC syndrome

Saethre-Chotzen syndrome: A rare genetic disorder characterized by craniosynostosis, acrocephaly and/or syndactyly. Craniofacial abnormalities may include ocular hypertelorism, shallow orbits, ptosis, strabismus, beak-like nose, deviated nasal septum, dysplastic ears, and hypoplastic maxilla. Other associated malformations may include cutaneous syndactyly, brachydactyly, and broad great toes. Some affected individuals may exhibit mild to moderate mental retardation, but normal intelligence is the normal situation.

Synonyms: ACS type III; ACS3; acrocephalosyndactyly type III; acrocephaly skull asymmetry and mild syndactyly; Chotzen syndrome; SCS

Toriello-Bauserman syndrome: An autosomal recessive disorder characterized by multiple ankyloses, camptodactyly, craniofacial anomalies, and pulmonary hypoplasia.

Velocardiofacial syndrome: *See* Conotruncal anomaly face syndrome.

von Voss syndrome: A rare, perinatally lethal, unusual complex of multiple congenital anomalies characterized by phocomelia, radial ray defects, hypomegakaryocytic thrombocytopenia, occipital encephalocele, and urogenital abnormalities.

Synonyms: von Voss-Cherstvoy syndrome; D K phocomelia syndrome

Zellweger syndrome: One of four diseases called *peroxisome biogenesis disorders* (PBD) within the category of leukodystrophies. Zellweger syndrome is an inherited condition that damages the white matter of the brain and affects how the body metabolizes particular substances in the blood and organ tissues. Symptoms resulting from high iron and copper serum concentrations include hepatomegaly, craniofacial deformities (high forehead, underdeveloped brow ridges, and dysplastic ears), mental retardation, and seizures.

REFERENCES

Benumof, J.L. (Ed.). (1998). *Anesthesia and Uncommon Diseases* (4th ed.). Philadelphia: Saunders.

Emedicine. Retrieved from www.emedicine.com

Fleisher, L.A. (Ed.). (2006). *Anesthesia and Uncommon Diseases* (5th ed.). Philadelphia: Saunders.

Stoelting, R.K., & Dierdorf, S.F. (Eds.). (2002). *Anesthesia and Co-Existing Diseases* (4th ed.). London: Churchill Livingstone.

INDEX

A

Accessory pathway ablation
    Lown-Ganong-Levine syndrome
        treated with, 197
    Wolff-Parkinson-White syndrome
        treated with, 357
Acetylcholine, 101-102
Acetylcholinesterase inhibitors,
    226-227
Achalasia
    anesthesia considerations, 3
    complications of, 3
    definition of, 1
    diagnosis of, 1-2
    etiology of, 1
    incidence of, 1
    pharmacologic treatment of, 1-2
    pneumatic catheter for, 2
    pneumonitis and, 3
    postoperative considerations, 3
    signs and symptoms of, 1
Achondroplasia
    atlantoaxial joint instability
        associated with, 7
    complications of, 6-8
    craniofacial anomalies in, 7
    definition of, 4
    etiology of, 4
    incidence of, 4
    laryngeal mask airway use in, 7
    laryngomalacia and, 7
    medical management of, 6
    regional anesthesia in, 7
    restrictive pulmonary disease in, 7
    signs and symptoms of, 4, 5f
    surgical treatment of, 6
Acromegaly
    anesthesia considerations, 11-12
    complications of, 11
    definition of, 9
    developmental sequence of, 10f
    etiology of, 9
    extubation considerations in, 12
    incidence of, 9
    medical management of, 11

Acromegaly *(Continued)*
    obstructive sleep apnea in, 12
    signs and symptoms of, 9-11
Actinomycin D. *See* Dactinomycin
Active zone particles, 101
Acute inflammatory demyelinating
    polyradiculoneuropathy. *See*
    Guillain-Barré syndrome
Acute leukemia
    anesthesia considerations, 15
    complications of, 15
    definition of, 13
    etiology of, 13
    incidence of, 13
    medical management of, 14
    signs and symptoms of, 14
Acute lymphocytic leukemia
    chemotherapy for, 15
    incidence of, 13
    medical management of, 15
Acute myelogenous leukemia
    incidence of, 13
    medical management of, 14
Acute porphyria
    anesthesia considerations for,
        18-21
    attack of, 19b, 20-21
    autonomic instability associated
        with, 18
    complications of, 18
    definition of, 16
    drugs that cause, 18b
    etiology of, 16
    general anesthesia for, 20
    incidence of, 16
    medical management of, 17-18,
        19b
    nausea and vomiting
        prevention, 21
    regional anesthesia for, 20
    signs and symptoms of, 17
    treatment of, 19b
    triggers for, 19b
    variants of, 16t

Page numbers followed by a b, indicate boxes; f, figures; t, tables.